NUTRITION AND LABORATORY MEDICINE

D1643212

Ruth Ayling PhD, MRCP, MRCPCH, FRCPath
Consultant Chemical Pathologist, Derriford Hospital NHS Trust, Plymouth

William Marshall PhD, FIBiol, FRCP, FRCPath, FRCPEdin
Clinical Director of Pathology, The London Clinic, London and Emeritus Reader in Clinical Biochemistry, King's College London

Foreword by Professor Alan Shenkin MB, ChB, PhD, FRCP, FRCPath

Editors:
Beverley Harris BSc, MSc, MRCPath
Principal Clinical Scientist, Royal United Hospital, Bath

Marta Lapsley MB, BCh, MD, MRCPath
Consultant Chemical Pathologist, Epsom Hospital, Surrey

ACB VENTURE PUBLICATIONS

ACB VENTURE PUBLICATIONS
Chairman - Ruth Lapworth

British Library Cataloguing in Publication Data

A catalogue record for the book is available from the British Library

ISBN 978-0-902429-44-4, EAN 9780902429444, ACB Venture Publications

Printed by Latimer Trends, Plymouth

Cover and illustrations by Alan Sherwood, Burnt Canvas Designs

Foreword

Over the past few years, nutrition has been increasingly recognised as of central importance, both to optimising health and to preventing and treating disease. On a public health basis, an inadequate or excessive diet may directly affect health, whereas in hospital care, adequate nutrition may be necessary not only to manage the consequences of a poor diet, but also to buy the time necessary for other forms of therapy to be effective.

One question which is frequently asked is how the laboratory should contribute to nutritional care. It is apparent that such care requires a multi-disciplinary approach. Although the doctor with primary responsibility for the patient is the leader of the team providing all aspects of care, he/she needs to make full use of all resources available – with respect to nutrition this is likely to include not only specialist nurses and dietitians, but also a wide range of other specialists with an appropriate interest. Clinical biochemistry based medical staff and clinical scientists are in a unique position to contribute in a supportive role, or indeed to take a lead role, depending upon their personal interest and whether there are other nutritional enthusiasts in their hospital.

A major problem in the development of services to provide nutritional therapy has been the fact that no medical specialty 'owns' nutrition. It is part of virtually all clinical specialties, to a greater or lesser extent being relevant to the aetiology and management of most disease states. This has led in the past to sporadic and often inconsistent training and knowledge of the principles and practice of nutritional therapy. More recently there have been some encouraging signs, with the development of the Intercollegiate Course on Human Nutrition, a course on the basic principles of nutrition that is attended by trainees from across the range of Medical Royal Colleges, and also the inclusion of basic nutritional care within the Foundation Programme for junior hospital doctors.

The lack of a 'home' for nutrition has, however, led to a gap in specialist competencies, which has been recognised by clinical biochemists. Doctors in hospitals, and those treating nutritional problems in primary care, welcome expert advice and comment from colleagues in clinical biochemistry who can advise them on investigation of nutritional problems and how to treat them. This in turn has been recognised by the training committees responsible for training clinical biochemists, both non-medical and medical, some of whom will also be training in the new clinical sub-specialty of metabolic medicine.

Appropriate nutritional care depends upon an accurate assessment of nutritional status, and of the nutritional and metabolic problems faced by a particular patient. This requires not only a thorough knowledge of nutritional requirements, but also an understanding of the pathophysiology of nutritional disorders – in other words the mechanisms by which a mismatch between metabolic demand and nutritional supply may occur, and the consequences of such a mismatch. With nutrition playing a variable part in undergraduate medical curricula, and specialist medical training being reduced often to the bare essentials, it becomes important that chemical pathologists and clinical scientists rise to the challenge of developing this expertise, so that they can contribute to this clinical understanding.

This book fills an important need in this area. Both by explaining the pathophysiology of nutritional disorders and the basics of nutritional care, it will make it possible for clinical biochemists to have the confidence to develop clinical experience in this field – by attending ward rounds, outpatient clinics or case review meetings – and hence develop the ability to make a valuable clinical contribution. Clinical nutrition is undoubtedly one of the best ways for a clinical biochemist to combine laboratory and clinical work, and to participate in education and research.

The authors are to be congratulated on a book which is both comprehensive and clearly written. It is especially useful that the subject areas include not only disease-related malnutrition and its management, but also diseases of overnutrition and a selection of disease-specific nutritional problems. Nutritional therapy is correctly expanded to include the common problems of fluid and electrolytes which frequently co-exist with protein-energy problems.

I am firmly of the belief that all Clinical Biochemistry Departments should ensure that at least one member of their staff, whether medically or scientifically qualified, picks up the challenge of contributing to nutritional care services within their hospital. They should ensure they can advise on the appropriate use of laboratory tests within the context of nutritional assessment, and have expertise in delivering and monitoring nutritional care. Although written by two experienced clinical biochemists, and primarily for clinical biochemists, this book will be of value to any specialist wishing to obtain an up-to-date grounding in clinical nutrition.

Alan Shenkin
University of Liverpool
June 2007

Preface

Adequate nutrition is central to the maintenance of health. Although undernutrition has obvious adverse effects, an excess of some nutrients, and particularly of overall energy intake, can be harmful. Nutritional disorders are common, but nutrition tends to be poorly represented in undergraduate medical and scientific curricula.

There are several reasons why nutrition is an important subject for clinical biochemists. Laboratory investigations are essential to the successful diagnosis and management of many nutritional disorders; nutritional disorders give rise to significant metabolic dysfunction, and clinical biochemists are frequently members of multidisciplinary teams advising on the provision of nutritional support.

In writing this book, we have attempted to bring together those aspects of nutrition that are particularly relevant to the clinical biochemist, whether scientifically or medically qualified. These include the functions of nutrients, the digestion and absorption of food, the assessment of nutritional status and the investigation and management of nutritional disorders, including both undernutrition and obesity.

We have enjoyed this collaboration, and are grateful to the ACB Venture Publications team for their encouragement throughout this project. Our especial thanks are due to Beverley Harris and Marta Lapsley for their patience, good humour and skill in editing our manuscript and managing us, and to Emma Woolman for so ably turning our Word files into printable format.

Ruth Ayling
William Marshall
Plymouth and London, June 2007

Contents

Chapter 1

The scope of clinical nutrition

Introduction

Adequate nutrition is essential for normal development, growth and function. Indeed, nutrition may be defined as the process whereby food substances are used for these purposes. Inadequate nutrition, for whatever reason it occurs, can have many harmful effects. Some of these are obvious, for example, the classic deficiency diseases which, although now rare in the so-called 'developed' world, remain a fact of life in many poorer countries (e.g. deficiency of vitamin A causes some 350,000 young children to become blind each year). Other effects are more subtle, for example, the effect of borderline iron deficiency, which may only become clinically apparent if an additional stress, such as pregnancy, is placed on the haemopoeitic system. Worldwide, it is estimated that more than 200 million children have sub-clinical deficiency of vitamin A and as a result have a higher incidence of severe infections and mortality than children with adequate vitamin A intakes. Generalised malnutrition is also a major problem and is estimated to be the cause of approximately half the annual 11 million deaths of children under the age of five.

Nutrition may be inadequate either because there is insufficient food (either in quality or quantity), or because the available food is not or cannot be consumed, or (more frequently) because there is impairment of the digestion, absorption or processing of its component nutrients. Most of the classic deficiency diseases, such as scurvy, rickets and pellagra, were described more than one hundred years ago, although the elucidation of their precise pathogenesis has depended on advances in biochemistry and physiology made mainly in the latter half of the last century. New physiological functions of vitamins are still being discovered, e.g. the role of vitamin D derivatives in cellular differentiation, as well as new therapeutic uses such as derivatives of vitamin D in myelodysplastic disorders.

More recently, the importance of excessive intake of food as a cause of disease has received considerable attention, for example, the links between a high intake of saturated fat, hypercholesterolaemia and coronary heart disease, and between a high intake of salt and hypertension. Indeed, many aspects of the modern 'Western diet', with its high content of protein and fat and relatively low content of unrefined carbohydrates and fibre compared with diets traditionally consumed in developing countries, have been identified as being potentially harmful, both to those for whom such a diet is usual and to those to whom it is introduced.

In many cases, nutritional disorders can be successfully treated by improvement or supplementation of the diet (provided that economic and other factors allow). However, for individuals who are unable for any reason to eat, digest or absorb food normally, nutrition may have to be maintained artificially rather than through the provision of adequate oral food intake.

The provision and maintenance of good nutrition is not only important in the prevention of disease; dietary manipulations also have an important role to play in the treatment of a wide variety of conditions, e.g. diabetes mellitus, renal disease, liver disease and many inherited metabolic diseases (see Chapter 7).

The study of nutrition embraces agricultural, economic, climatic, geographical, cultural, sociological, political and religious issues (all of which, though important, are beyond the scope of this book), as well as physiology and biochemistry. Whereas the latter have provided us with much of the rational basis for our understanding of the role of nutrients at a cellular and molecular level, the applied branches of these sciences, notably clinical physiology and clinical biochemistry, provide us with many of the techniques of nutritional assessment that are essential for the successful practice of clinical nutrition.

Clinical nutrition has been, and continues to be, a neglected aspect of medical practice. It has often been accorded little space in undergraduate medical curricula in the UK despite various initiatives for change, including the publication of a core curriculum for nutrition by the Department of Health as part of the 'Health of the Nation' strategy. Nutrition has not hitherto been regarded as a distinct medical specialty with defined postgraduate training, although it is relevant to all medical practitioners. However, nutrition is part of the curriculum of training in metabolic medicine in the UK, for which there are now joint training schemes in both general internal medicine and chemical pathology. Also, in England and Wales, the National Institute for Health and Clinical Excellence (NICE) has published comprehensive (and, where possible, evidence based) guidelines for nutrition support in adults (see Further Reading). These include recommendations on screening, diagnosis and management. It is to be hoped that the promulgation of these guidelines will increase healthcare professionals' awareness of the importance of nutrition and, with time, reduce the prevalence of undernutrition in patients in hospitals and the community and in the residents of care homes.

Dietitians have a pivotal role in clinical nutrition but other healthcare professionals are becoming increasingly involved. These include clinical biochemists (both scientifically and medically trained), nurses, pharmacists and doctors in medical and surgical specialties. Parents and teachers also have key roles to play.

While the content of this book primarily examines the interface between clinical nutrition and laboratory medicine, we attempt to do this in the context of clinical nutrition as a whole.

In this chapter, we survey some of the conditions that result from inappropriate nutrition or that respond to nutritional intervention. Later chapters expand on some of these and examine the absorption of nutrients and their cellular and molecular roles; the assessment of nutritional status; the provision of nutrition support; the role of nutritional manipulations in conditions that are not primarily of nutritional origin and the use of nutrients other than to maintain normal structure and function. Obesity is accorded a chapter of its own.

Nutrients: an overview

Nutrients can be classified into sources of energy (primarily fats and carbohydrates), sources of nitrogen (proteins), major minerals (sodium, potassium etc.) and micronutrients (trace elements and vitamins). Energy can also be obtained by oxidation of the carbon skeletons of amino acids, although with most diets protein is only a minor energy source. The maintenance of body temperature is a major drain on the body's energy supplies. Absorption of heat energy from the surroundings can reduce this, but such energy is not available directly to the body for other purposes.

Many components of the diet require considerable processing to make the nutrients that they contain available to the body's tissues. Digestion and absorption are major stages of this process, but metabolism, particularly in the liver, is also important.

Food also contains substances with no nutrient value in classic terms, some of which appear to be beneficial (e.g. certain dietary fibres, naturally occurring antioxidants) while others are potentially harmful (e.g. fungal toxins) or are inconsequential in the amounts normally consumed. Food almost invariably contains substances that are added in the course of production, for example hormones given to animals as growth supplements, fungicides used on vegetable and fruit crops, and preservatives and additives used in manufactured foods to enhance palatability, shelf life or physical appearance.

There is growing interest in the use of food to promote (rather than maintain) health. This includes the use of supplements of biologically active substances, e.g. amino acids (sometimes referred to as 'nutraceuticals'), and the use of 'probiotics' – live, supposedly beneficial, bacteria. This area has attracted much interest from practitioners of complementary medicine but it is likely that it will become increasingly subject to scientific scrutiny and, if proven to be of benefit, become adopted into conventional medical practice. The development of nutritional genomics – genetic analysis aimed at defining the genetic factors in individuals that determine intraindividual response to nutrients – may provide some stimulus to this process.

Disorders of deficit

Normal adaptation to starvation

If energy intake is less than the body's requirements, there will be a net negative energy balance. Since the body's reserves of carbohydrate (mainly hepatic glycogen; glycogen in muscle can supply energy only to muscle) are sufficient for only about 18 h of normal expenditure, energy deficits must be met by the mobilisation of fat. During fasting, adaptive changes take place to minimise the body's requirements for glucose. Some tissues (e.g. red blood cells) have an absolute requirement for glucose as their source of energy. The brain, however, although normally dependent on glucose, can adapt to utilise ketone bodies derived from fat. Skeletal muscle can utilise glucose, free fatty acids and ketones. Thus, although the requirement for glucose as an energy source decreases during prolonged fasting, some glucose is still required and, since it cannot be synthesised from fat, must be supplied by gluconeogenesis. This is the synthesis of glucose primarily from the carbon skeletons of amino acids and to a lesser extent from the glycerol that is released during the hydrolysis of triacylglycerols.

Adjustment of energy intake such that it is sustained at less than output is the basis of the treatment of obesity. In non-obese individuals, however, persistently inadequate energy intake leads to wasting of fat and lean body mass. Severe starvation is frequently complicated by infection: gastrointestinal infection may cause diarrhoea and further compromise nutrition. Starvation in adults leads to generalised wasting and increasing functional disturbance. In children, however, two major clinical syndromes are recognised: marasmus and kwashiorkor.

Generalised malnutrition: starvation, marasmus and kwashiorkor

In marasmus, there is severe, generalised wasting, with loss of body fat and muscle. The facial appearance is that of an old person but, in contrast to kwashiorkor, there is no oedema. The etymology is from a Greek word meaning 'a dying away'. It is common in all areas where starvation is endemic and is familiar to people in other places through television and newspaper reports. Although the term is applied to children, starvation in adults has similar consequences and can be seen in Western countries in patients with severe anorexia nervosa or intestinal failure.

Plasma insulin concentrations are low in marasmus and those of cortisol are increased. This leads to the breakdown of muscle protein to provide a fuel for gluconeogenesis. However, hepatic albumin synthesis is relatively well preserved so that, despite severe muscle wasting, plasma albumin concentrations are usually normal in the early stages of marasmus and there is no peripheral oedema.

Wasting also occurs with kwashiorkor but may not be so obvious owing to the oedema and abdominal ascites that characterise this condition. The term 'oedematous malnutrition' is now recommended but 'kwashiorkor' is still widely used. It was first described in Ghana (then called the Gold Coast) and was observed to occur in children who were displaced from the breast following the birth of a younger sibling. It has generally been supposed to be due to a deficiency of protein with adequate energy intake. Plasma insulin concentrations are higher and plasma cortisol concentrations lower than in marasmus. As a result, hepatic albumin synthesis is decreased, leading to hypoalbuminaemia and, it has been supposed, to the characteristic peripheral oedema and abdominal ascites. However, some studies have shown no difference between the protein intakes of children with oedema and those without, and other factors are certainly involved. These may include infection, potassium depletion (leading to sodium retention) and specific dietary deficiencies (e.g. of trace elements, sulphur-containing amino acids and vitamins C and E), which lead to impairment of the body's free radical scavenging mechanisms. Plasma concentrations of glutathione are reduced in this condition and the highest mortality is associated with the most marked decreases in the activity of glutathione peroxidase. However, a recent clinical trial of anti-oxidant supplementation did not reduce the development of kwashiorkor in a group of children at high risk. It has also been suggested that kwashiorkor represents a failure of adaptation to starvation. Other features of the condition include fatty infiltration of the liver, which may cause hepatomegaly and is thought to be due to decreased apolipoprotein synthesis. A similar clinical picture to kwashiorkor has occasionally been observed in human adults deprived of protein but having an adequate energy intake.

Infection is a frequent consequence of generalised malnutrition. Many factors are involved, including decreased production of immunoglobulins as a result of reduced protein synthesis, a decrease in the number of T lymphocytes, decreased lymphocyte function, impaired phagocytosis and a decrease in secretory IgA. Loss of delayed hypersensitivity is frequently present, and has been used as a test for nutritional status. There is decreased function of most of the body's organ systems: even though the brain's function tends to be relatively preserved, a flattening of affect with apathy or depression is frequent.

Stunting of growth is characteristic of malnutrition. Although mainly seen in countries where malnutrition is endemic, it can occur in developed countries owing to generalised malabsorption, e.g. due to coeliac disease, as well as in conditions such as chronic infection, chronic renal disease and hypothyroidism. The mean height of adults has increased in the UK over the centuries and this is thought to be a result of improved nutrition and decreased infection.

It must be emphasised that marasmus and kwashiorkor are the severest manifestations of malnutrition. In areas where malnutrition is endemic, far more children will suffer growth retardation and are at increased risk of infection than develop clinical marasmus or kwashiorkor.

The management of these conditions is in theory straightforward: provision of a qualitatively and quantitatively adequate food intake. If there are no complicating circumstances, e.g. infection, disruption of mucous membranes or organ failure, this should restore nutrition and health. In practice, it is often far from straightforward and in some areas of the world malnutrition appears to be an intractable problem.

The primary objective of treatment might appear to be correction of the weight loss by immediate provision of large amounts of nutrients. This is potentially very dangerous. Severe malnutrition may be complicated by hypothermia, hypoglycaemia, fluid and electrolyte disturbances and infection. If any of these is present, appropriate resuscitative measures will be required. Refeeding must be commenced gradually, initially giving only a quarter of estimated nitrogen and energy requirements but full replacement of minerals and vitamins, and increasing the nitrogen and energy intake to full requirements by the end of the first week. If refeeding is not begun gradually in this way, dangerous metabolic imbalances, particularly hypokalaemia and hypophosphataemia, and fluid retention leading to cardiac failure, may occur. This is a consequence of the provision of energy in the face of continuing deficits of vital nutrients, stimulating metabolism that has become adapted to a low nutrient intake.

The management of generalised malnutrition in countries where the majority of the population is adequately nourished (including the avoidance of the refeeding syndrome), is considered further in Chapter 5.

Anorexia nervosa and bulimia nervosa

It is outside the scope of this book to discuss the pathogenesis of these eating disorders in detail and the interested reader is referred to reviews listed under Further Reading at the end of the chapter. Many factors – social, cultural, familial and genetic – may be involved. Both conditions are commoner in females than males and the risk of eating disorders is increased ten-fold in first degree relatives of individuals with anorexia nervosa. There may be a family or personal history of obsessive-compulsive disorder.

Anorexia nervosa is characterised by a persistent failure of the sufferer to eat sufficient to maintain an appropriate body weight for his or her height (more than 85% of ideal body weight or body mass index (BMI) greater than 17.5 kg/m^2). Patients are frequently preoccupied with their weight, perceive themselves as being fat when they are not and have an intense fear of gaining weight. The condition is potentially fatal. Presentation is usually with cachexia, amenorrhoea and often postural hypotension as a result of a low plasma volume, with bradycardia. The low plasma volume may cause a mild pre-renal uraemia. Specific nutrient deficiencies are uncommon: patients often eat adequate protein and micronutrients. Iron deficiency may occur but is uncommon, as most patients do not menstruate. Fine lanugo hair may grow on the cheeks, forearms and thighs. The diagnosis is usually obvious from the history and evidence of weight loss but it may be necessary to exclude other conditions that can cause weight loss (e.g. thyrotoxicosis) or amenorrhoea (e.g. primary ovarian failure).

The amenorrhoea is associated with decreased plasma concentrations of gonadotrophins; if this persists, it predisposes to osteoporosis. This, and the clinical features, may suggest a diagnosis of hypopituitarism, but other features of this condition are not present: plasma cortisol concentrations are typically elevated in anorexia nervosa and may not be suppressible by dexamethasone. The weight loss in anorexia nervosa is usually more marked than is typical of hypopituitarism.

The management of anorexia nervosa requires the combined skills of a psychiatrist and a dietitian, supported by nurses, therapists and other staff. However, the condition often recurs and the prognosis is poor. Artificial nutrition support is not recommended but may occasionally be required if a patient develops severe complications, e.g. renal failure. Refeeding requires close supervision to avoid the refeeding syndrome, characterised by electrolyte disturbances (e.g. hypokalaemia, hypomagnesaemia, hypocalcaemia, hypophosphataemia) and a risk of acute gastric dilatation. The lower the BMI, the greater is the risk. Similar problems can occur in individuals who binge and purge.

Bulimia nervosa is a separate condition, though it can occur in conjunction with anorexia nervosa or follow it. There is binge eating associated with self-induced vomiting, purging or avoidance of food. Weight loss is generally less severe than in anorexia (some patients have normal or even increased body weight), as are the endocrine changes. Three physical signs are characteristic: trauma to the skin on the dorsum of the hands overlying the metacarpophalangeal joints (secondary to self-induced vomiting), salivary gland hyperplasia and dental erosions due to repeated exposure of the teeth to acidic gastric juice. Loss of gastric acid can cause metabolic alkalosis whereas laxative abuse can lead to excess loss of bicarbonate in the stools and metabolic acidosis.

The management of bulimia is as challenging as that of anorexia. Other psychiatric disorders may coexist with both conditions.

Specific deficiencies

Disorders due to specific nutrient deficiencies may be seen in individuals suffering from generalised malnutrition, but can also occur in isolation. Most are rare in developed countries, exceptions being osteomalacia and rickets (caused by deficiency of vitamin D), and nutritional anaemias (due to deficiencies of iron, folic acid or vitamin B_{12}). Deficiencies of other nutrients may occur in particularly susceptible individuals. Specific deficiencies are discussed in detail in Chapter 2.

Nutritional consequences of non-gastrointestinal disease

Although it is readily understandable that patients with disease involving the gastrointestinal tract and its associated organs are at risk of becoming undernourished, nutritional depletion is a frequent consequence of illness in general. Although the factors responsible may be different, there is often a final common pathway involving decreased food intake (particularly because of decreased appetite) and increased energy expenditure. As is discussed in Chapter 5, nutritional depletion can itself have adverse consequences on disease outcome, for example by predisposing to infection, impairing the activity of the immune system and delaying wound healing.

Cancer cachexia

Weight loss is a common feature of cancer, typically affecting more than 50% of patients and often being the presenting feature or a major manifestation of the condition. The mechanisms involved are complex, but the production of cytokines, particularly tumour necrosis factor alpha (TNFα), is frequently implicated. These induce a catabolic state and cause anorexia. Treatment with chemotherapy and radiotherapy may cause nausea, vomiting and diarrhoea. Associated depression may further decrease appetite. In gastrointestinal malignancies, physical obstruction to the gut may be an important contributory factor.

The management of cancer cachexia requires a team approach. Even patients within weeks of dying may benefit from intervention in terms of improved mood and appetite. Dietary measures include the provision of small, frequent, easily eaten and pleasant-tasting, energy-dense meals or dietary supplements. If early satiety is a problem, prokinetic agents (e.g. metoclopramide) may be of value; progestagens such as medroxyprogesterone can increase appetite and improve food intake but increase body fat rather than muscle. Anabolic steroids may have a place in the treatment of some patients. Measures to reduce inflammation may also be beneficial. Many possible treatments are currently being evaluated, but the heterogeneity of patients is only one of several factors that hamper the design of clinical trials.

Cardiac cachexia

Weight is a poor guide to nutritional status in patients with cardiac failure because of the tendency to retain fluid and the effects of diuretics used in treatment. These may disguise the loss of fat and lean body mass that is frequently present and is a poor prognostic sign. The precise mechanisms are unclear but probably involve neuroendocrine responses to alterations in tissue perfusion.

Chronic renal failure

The nutritional management of patients with chronic renal failure requires considerable skill. On the one hand, there is a need to restrict protein intake (although not as rigorously as used to be recommended) in order to reduce the load on the kidneys; on the other, the need to minimise the effect on nitrogen balance. The uraemic state is itself a catabolic state as a result of factors including the systemic acidosis and altered endocrine milieu. Renal replacement therapy, particularly continuous ambulatory peritoneal dialysis and haemofiltration techniques, can lead to loss of small molecular weight nutrients.

Chronic liver disease

As with cardiac failure, weight is often a misleading guide to nutritional status in chronic liver disease. Loss of fat and lean body mass is common and is multifactorial: decreased dietary protein intake (both prescribed as part of the management of encephalopathy and involuntary due to anorexia, nausea and the physical effect of ascites); alterations in metabolism; cholestasis, and associated pancreatic insufficiency (in alcohol-related liver disease) may all contribute.

Respiratory disorders

Maintaining adequate nutrition in patients with cystic fibrosis (particularly in children, in whom requirements are high because of the demands of growth) is a considerable challenge, but improvements in nutrition have undoubtedly improved the prognosis for people with this condition. Contributory factors have included the use of pancreatic enzyme supplementation and more effective treatment and prevention of pulmonary disease.

It is less often appreciated that patients with chronic obstructive pulmonary disease are at risk of becoming malnourished and the relatively recent recognition of this fact has led to improvements in pulmonary rehabilitation regimens and prognosis. Factors responsible include: the increased energy costs of breathing; breathlessness induced by eating resulting in decreased food intake; the energy costs of the skeletal (quadriceps) myopathy that is present in a high proportion of patients with chronic obstructive pulmonary disease; infection, and downwards pressure on the abdomen from hyperinflated lungs.

Connective tissue disorders
Muscle wasting is common in rheumatoid arthritis and other connective tissue disorders. This may be in part a direct result of decreased use of muscles responsible for the movement of affected joints, but the major factor is thought to be increased secretion of TNFα.

Other conditions
Many other conditions are associated with weight loss. In type 1 diabetes, thyrotoxicosis and primary adrenal failure it is often a presenting feature, but is rapidly reversed by effective treatment. The same applies to tuberculosis. It used to be a major feature of HIV infection but is now less of a problem in countries where highly active antiretroviral therapy is available: it is still a huge problem in the poorer countries of the world. In any illness, particularly if chronic or potentially terminal, the presence of depression may suppress appetite and further compromise nutrition.

Management
The development and application of effective strategies for the prevention and treatment of disease-associated malnutrition depends first on recognition of the problem. Questions about food intake and weight loss should be a standard component of history-taking and measurements of nutritional status should be made as part of the clinical examination in all patients. In England and Wales, the National Institute for Health and Clinical Excellence (NICE) recommends that all hospital inpatients and outpatients are screened at their first encounter (and at intervals thereafter) using the Malnutrition Universal Screening Tool (MUST). Impediments to adequate nutrition (e.g. anorectic drugs, depression) must be recognised and managed appropriately. The input of a dietitian is essential, both to advise on an appropriate regimen of nutritional supplementation and to monitor the response to treatment. There is encouraging evidence that in some conditions such interventions have a positive effect on outcome, but they must be part of an overall programme of non-medical management, including, for example, graded exercise.

There is considerable ongoing research into the use of pharmacological interventions to reduce catabolism and improve food intake. The recent elucidation of the endocrine mechanisms involved in hunger and satiety may provide the basis for significant advances in this field (see Chapter 6).

Disorders of excess

Obesity
Obesity is the commonest nutritional disorder seen in developed countries. It is often defined in relation to the body mass index (BMI, also known as Quetelet's index after the Belgian astronomer and polymath who first described it). The BMI is calculated as the individual's weight (kg) divided by the square of their height (m). Values of 19-24.9 kg/m^2 are considered normal and are associated with the lowest mortality. Individuals with values in the range 25-29.9 are classified as overweight; a value over 30 classifies the individual as obese. Data for England and Wales in 2000 indicated that more than 21% of men and women were obese and over 50% were overweight. These figures compare with less than 10% for obesity in 1980. The prevalence of obesity is increasing worldwide, particularly in developing countries. It is a particular concern that the prevalence of obesity is increasing in children as well as in adults. Between 1995 and 2003 the prevalence of obesity in children in the UK aged 2-10 years increased from 9.9% to 13.7%. In 2003, over 25% of children in this age group were overweight. Obesity is a major risk factor for type 2 diabetes (and hence for cardiovascular disease) and is associated with an increased risk of many other conditions. Whereas type 2 diabetes used to be considered a disease of middle and late life, it is now being diagnosed with increasing frequency in children, giving rise to the suggestion that a significant number of children in the current generation will be outlived by their parents.

Major advances have occurred in our understanding of the pathogenesis of obesity in recent years, coupled with an appreciation that adipocytes are not just cells that store fat but are metabolically highly active, responding to and secreting hormones and cytokines. It has also become apparent that the cardiovascular complications of obesity depend on the distribution of the excess fat: they are more likely to occur with abdominal rather than gluteal adiposity, that is, when the waist-hip ratio (the ratio of girth at the waist to that measured round the hips) exceeds 1.0 in men and 0.8 in women.

The pathogenesis, consequences and management of obesity are discussed in detail in Chapter 6.

Type 2 diabetes mellitus
This is a multifactorial condition. There is a strong genetic component with over 90% concordance for the development of type 2 diabetes between monozygotic (genetically identical) twins.

However, as alluded to above, being overweight is a major risk factor for diabetes, some 80% of patients with the condition being overweight. As is discussed in a later chapter (p.179), dietary modification is an essential part of the management of type 2 diabetes; if overweight patients are able to reduce their weight to an appropriate value for their height, their glucose tolerance may be greatly improved.

Cardiovascular disease
There are numerous risk factors for cardiovascular, cerebrovascular and peripheral vascular disease. The most important include dyslipidaemias (particularly hypercholesterolaemia and, specifically, increased plasma LDL cholesterol concentrations), cigarette smoking, hypertension and type 2 diabetes. Hypercholesterolaemia can be inherited or acquired. Dietary cholesterol intake correlates poorly with plasma cholesterol concentration (the major determinant of which is the relative rates of hepatic synthesis and clearance), but there is a strong correlation with the dietary intake of saturated fats. Dietary modification is the cornerstone of the management of the dyslipidaemias and is discussed in greater detail in a later chapter (p.177). It must be stressed, however, that the approach to the management and prevention of cardiovascular disease must embrace all the identifiable risk factors. Many patients will require drug treatment as well as dietary modification and other lifestyle changes.

There are many other associations between diet and cardiovascular disease. The risk of cardiovascular disease is negatively correlated with fruit, vegetable and wholegrain cereal consumption. This has been supposed to be related to the antioxidant content of these foods, but this notion has not been supported by the results of secondary prevention trials: supplementation of the diet with vitamins C and E and β-carotene have not been shown to affect either the risk of further cardiovascular events or overall mortality. However, green vegetables are a good source of folic acid, and dietary folate supplementation has been shown to lower plasma homocysteine concentrations; hyperhomocysteinaemia is a recognised risk factor for cardiovascular disease. Unfortunately, the evidence that folate supplementation has a beneficial effect on cardiovascular disease is inconsistent.

Hypertension
Hypertension is a common condition. Most patients with hypertension are asymptomatic but there is an increased risk of coronary heart disease, stroke and

renal disease. Whereas recognised causes of hypertension (e.g. renal disease and hypersecretion of adrenal steroids) can sometimes be identified, most (approximately 90%) hypertension is 'essential' and the precise cause is unknown. Genetic and dietary factors are known to be important. There are positive correlations between sodium intake, alcohol intake, obesity and hypertension, and a negative correlation with potassium intake.

It is beyond the scope of this book to review the extensive and, at times, contradictory literature on salt and hypertension. Most people in developed countries have a higher sodium intake than the body requires (often considerably higher). The kidneys are very efficient at conserving sodium and the obligatory renal sodium loss in normal individuals is less than 20 mmol/24 h, yet the average daily sodium intake in the UK is at least four times this. The evidence in favour of a link between mean dietary sodium intake and the prevalence of hypertension (the 'salt hypothesis') can be summarised as follows:

- comparing the populations of countries, there is a positive correlation between mean dietary salt intake and the prevalence of hypertension
- reduction of salt intake in individuals with hypertension usually results in a decrease in blood pressure (albeit often modest)
- blood pressure tends to increase if salt intake is increased above the normal for an individual.

This is strong evidence and is considered by most physicians to be a justification for recommending a decrease in salt intake in patients with hypertension. However, it has not been possible to demonstrate a consistent correlation between salt intake and blood pressure in individuals, other than those with a family history of hypertension (in whom such a correlation has been demonstrated). The evidence also suggests that benefit should accrue were the mean salt intake of the population to be reduced. This is an important public health issue and there are currently several initiatives aimed at doing this, both through persuading manufacturers to add less salt to foods and through education of the public.

Some individuals with hypertension appear to respond to a decrease in dietary salt intake to a greater extent than others. Given the high intake of many people, a reduction is usually fairly easy to achieve and may be sufficient to avoid treatment with hypotensive drugs (many of which have side effects) or to allow effective control of blood pressure at a lower dosage. The mechanism linking dietary salt and hypertension is unclear, but patients with hypertension have been shown to have a tendency to accumulate intracellular sodium (which may increase the tone of arteriolar smooth muscle cells and hence increase peripheral resistance) and this may be exacerbated by a high sodium intake.

Alcohol

Excessive consumption of alcohol (ethanol) has many deleterious effects, most of which lie outside the scope of this book. In addition to liver disease in susceptible individuals, it increases the risk of cardiomyopathy, skeletal myopathy, osteo-porosis, pancreatitis, stroke and some malignancies. It is also a potential risk factor for obesity, 1 g of alcohol having an energy equivalent of 7 kcal (~29 kJoules). However, the potential is offset in some individuals by virtue of their having a poor overall nutrient intake and hence energy from more conventional sources. They may also be at risk of deficiency of certain B vitamins such as niacin, thiamin and pyridoxine. Some alcoholic beverages contain substances that may be beneficial: for example, red wine is relatively rich in antioxidants and this may to some extent explain the apparent protective effect of a moderate intake of alcohol as red wine against coronary heart disease and some cancers.

Cancer

Numerous cancers show an association with excess intake of certain nutrients, although there are also examples of nutrients that can reduce the risk of tumours. In most cases, however, there is no evidence of causation. For example, although epidemiological data indicate that a high fat intake increases the risk of breast cancer in post-menopausal women, this is not supported by the results of prospective studies. In the few instances where causation has been clearly proven, the agent responsible has been shown to be a contaminant of food. Examples include aflatoxin, produced by mould growing on peanuts (cancers of the oesoph-agus, stomach and liver) and polycylic hydrocarbons that have been reported to be generated by some smoking procedures used to 'cure' fish and meat (stomach).

On the other hand, there is considerable evidence of benefit from certain dietary components as far as the risk of cancer is concerned. A high intake of fibre, for example, appears to reduce the risk of colorectal cancer.

Other harmful effects of food

As has already been indicated, the potential harmful effects of some foods are not limited to the disorders of excess that have been described above. Foods may naturally contain potentially harmful substances but in quantities that are insuffi-cient to cause harm (e.g. oxalate in spinach and rhubarb) or cause harm only in susceptible individuals (see 'Food sensitivity', p.15). It may become contaminated either during production (e.g. fruit with insecticides, meat with antibiotics or hormones) or owing to spoilage (e.g. solanine, a toxic alkaloid that is formed in green potatoes). Food poisoning by microorganisms is discussed briefly on p.16. There is presently considerable concern that genetic modification of foodstuffs may be potentially harmful, both to the environment and to consumers. Some genetic modifications are designed to improve nutrient value but others to increase yields (for example, by making a crop resistant to a herbicide that can be used to control competing weeds) and the concern is that the engineered genes may escape into neighbouring crops or natural vegetation.

Substances added to foods, either as preservatives or to enhance flavour, texture or visual appeal, may also be harmful to certain individuals and this topic is one of considerable current public interest. A less well recognised problem is the possible harmful effects of supplementing the diet with known nutrients. A considerable number of so-called 'natural' products are available, particularly in health food shops, and while most are harmless, this cannot always be assumed to be the case. The toxic effects of vitamin A are well known; vitamin D is also toxic in excess and even water soluble vitamins, any excess of which it might be assumed would be excreted in the urine, are not completely harmless. For example, an intake of pyridoxine (vitamin B_6) of 200 mg daily (admittedly some seventy times normal requirements) can cause neuropathy. Dietary supplements of calcium and vitamin D may be of value in preventing osteoporosis, but may cause hypercalciuria and predispose to urinary calculi.

In patients fed artificially, the potential to do harm by giving nutrients in excess is considerable. It is well recognised that the provision of energy substrates in excess of the body's ability to utilise them during parenteral nutrition is one of the factors that can lead to the hepatic dysfunction that can complicate this process (see p.152). Plasma concentrations of manganese in the potentially toxic range have been demonstrated in children on parenteral feeding given supposedly normal daily requirements of this element (see p.51).

Food sensitivity

This term encompasses a spectrum of conditions ranging from true intolerance, e.g. of lactose in individuals with lactase deficiency, through sensitivity that has a clear immunological basis, e.g. coeliac disease, to true allergies. The latter occur in 2-6% of the population in the UK. The manifestations of food allergy include vomiting, urticaria, bronchospasm, angioedema and, rarely, potentially fatal anaphylaxis. Milk, eggs, nuts and shellfish appear to be the most common culprits. In most such cases, it is possible to demonstrate hypersensitivity to an allergen using skin testing or RAST (radioallergosorbent test) testing to detect specific IgE. The presence of a positive test to an allergen does not necessarily mean that the individual will be clinically allergic, nor does the titre predict the severity of an allergic response. However, a negative test is good evidence that an apparently allergic reaction to the foodstuff is not mediated by IgE. In children, and to a lesser extent in adults, food sensitivity may also be associated with eczema (in early childhood) and asthma (typically after the age of five years), and skin testing may be positive. In some individuals, despite clear clinical evidence of sensitivity to a component of the diet, no immunological abnormality can be demonstrated. Individuals who have true food allergies and who have experienced severe reactions should carry a self-injecting device containing epinephrine (adrenaline).

Food sensitivity is treated by identification of the offending foodstuff and its elimination from the diet. If the association is clear this may be straightforward, but when it is not the process may be a long one. Adequate labelling of food is important, but even then it may not be readily apparent that a food item contains something to which an individual is sensitive if it is present as a derivative, e.g. nut oil.

A food sensitivity of particular interest to clinical biochemists is favism (haemolytic anaemia after eating fava beans), which is caused by glucose 6-phosphate dehydrogenase deficiency. Lactase deficiency and coeliac disease are discussed elsewhere in this book (pp.99 and 97, respectively).

Food hygiene and food poisoning

One of the great advances in public health in the 20th century has been improvement in standards of food processing hygiene, including every step from sourcing to consumption. However, this has not been achieved without raising some concerns, for example, in relation to the use of preservatives (and other additives) and to the potential for loss of nutrients during processing and cooking.

Food poisoning continues to be a frequent source of time off work in the UK but can have more severe consequences in the elderly and debilitated or in other groups (e.g. *Listeria monocytogenes* in pregnant women). According to the organism, the clinical illness can be due to either an exotoxin, produced in the food before ingestion (typically having a rapid onset) or an endotoxin, produced by bacterial multiplication in the gut; some (e.g. *Bacillus cereus*) can produce both. However, a detailed discussion of the different microorganisms that can cause food poisoning is beyond the scope of this book and so this topic will not be considered further here.

Food and drugs

Drugs and food can interact in several ways. For example, the bioavailability of many drugs taken orally is affected by whether they are taken before, with or after meals. Their metabolism can also be affected by food: grapefruit juice inhibits the cytochrome P450 CYP3A4 enzyme that is responsible for metabolising many drugs.

Drugs can also interfere with nutrition, by suppressing or enhancing appetite or through effects on metabolism (e.g. the catabolic effect of glucocorticoids and reduction of circulating 25-hydroxycholecalciferol concentrations by certain anti-convulsants). This is a complex area, and the interested reader should consult the Further Reading for more information.

Conclusion

Nutrition is a fundamental basic and clinical science. Laboratory scientists may be involved in various aspects, particularly in the diagnosis and management of nutritional disorders. Nutrition shares with laboratory medicine, and clinical biochemistry in particular, the distinction of being of relevance to every medical specialty.

Further reading

Ciliberto H, Ciliberto M, Briend A, Ashorn P, Bier D, Manary M. Antioxidant supplementation for the prevention of kwashiorkor in Malawian children; randomised, double blind, placebo controlled trial. Brit Med J 2005; **330**: 1109. (*see also Leading article in same issue:* Fuchs GJ. Antioxidants for children with kwashiorkor. Brit Med J 2005; **330**: 1095-1096).

Elliott R, Ong TJ. Nutritional genomics. Brit Med J 2002; **324:** 1438-1432.

Fearon KCH, Moses AGW. Cancer cachexia. Int J Cardiol 2002; **85**: 73-81. *Note: this issue (1 September) of Volume 85 (pp 1-191), is devoted entirely to cachexia and chronic illness.*

McNeill G, Cummings JH. Nutrition and common health problems. Clin Med 2004; **4**: 400-404.

National Institute for Health and Clinical Excellence 2006. Nutrition support in adults (www.nice.org.uk/page.aspx?o=cg032fullguideline).

Shetty P. Malnutrition and undernutrition. Medicine 2003; **31**: 18-22.

Stice E. Risk and maintenance factors for eating pathology: a meta-analytic review. Psychol Bull 2002; **128**: 825-848.

Treasure J. Eating disorders. Medicine 2004; **32**: 63-66.

Truswell AS. Diet-drug interactions. In: Garrow JS, James WP, Ralph A (Eds). Human Nutrition and Dietetics (10th edition), Edinburgh: Churchill Livingstone, 2000 pp. 829-836.

Truswell AS. Food sensitivity. In: Truswell AS. ABC of Nutrition (4th edition). London: BMA Books, 2003, pp 108-112.

Chapter 2

The biochemistry and physiology of individual nutrients

Introduction

Nutrients – components of the diet that are essential for health – can be classified in various ways. One is to divide them into macro- and micronutrients, on the basis of the quantities that are required to maintain healthy structure and function, but this is somewhat arbitrary and the amount of a substance that is required has no bearing on its essential nature. Nutrients can also be classified on the basis of their chemical nature, for example, carbohydrates, proteins, fats and minerals, and a fifth group, the vitamins, which is chemically diverse and includes simple molecules, such as ascorbic acid, as well as complex ones, such as vitamin B_{12}.

In this chapter, we divide nutrients into energy sources (principally carbohydrate and fat), proteins, minerals and vitamins (many of which are cofactors, or precursors of cofactors, for enzymes). We also include non-nutrient components of the diet (e.g. non-digestible vegetable fibres) and water, which although often not considered as a nutrient, is essential for life (in the short term to a far greater extent than any other component of the diet). Xenobiotics (substances naturally present in or added to food that do not contribute usefully to metabolic function) and nutraceuticals (nutrients that are added to the diet in supraphysiological amounts and other, non-essential substances, added to the diet for pharmacological purposes) are considered in Chapter 7.

Various terms are used to describe ideal nutrient intakes, for example, the RDI (recommended daily intake), which is the average intake that should meet the needs of most members of the population, and the LRNI (lower reference nutrient intake), which defines the needs of 95% of the population. Recommendations may vary between countries, and the optimum intake of many nutrients is dependent on age, sex, physiological variables and in some cases the intake of other nutrients. The figures provided in this chapter are intended only to be indicative, and should not be used on their own in the management of individual patients.

For each nutrient, we describe its function, dietary sources, homeostasis, clinical consequences of deficiency (and, where relevant, excess) and assessment of status.

CHAPTER 2

Major organic nutrients and water

Water

FUNCTION

All body fluids are aqueous solutions and though some organisms can survive periods of dessication, most cannot. Water is also required to allow the excretion of waste products in urine; obligatory loss in urine and, to a lesser extent, from the skin, lungs and in faeces (the first two comprising 'insensible' losses) continues even if no water is consumed. In a previously healthy individual, even if obligatory losses are as low as possible, complete water deprivation usually causes death within 7-10 days, and severe functional deficit long before that. If insensible losses are greater (e.g. because of high body or ambient temperature increasing sweating), this period can be much reduced. On a normal diet, given minimum insensible losses, the essential water requirement is approximately 1 mL/kg body weight/24 h. The figure is greater in children, in whom the body surface area to weight ratio is greater, and who thus have greater insensible water losses; it is higher still in the newborn, in whom the ability of the kidneys to conserve water is less than in adults, and highest in premature infants because of their poorly keratinised skin. The latent heat required to evaporate the water in sweat is an important factor in the control of body temperature: insensible water (and sodium) losses can be considerably increased in hot climates and with exercise.

SOURCES

Small amounts of water (approximately 300 mL/24 h) are produced from oxidative metabolism when hydrogen is oxidised to water. This amount is increased in catabolic individuals and may make a significant contribution to body water status in patients with acute renal failure.

Most foodstuffs contain water and for most individuals in developed countries, water and other fluids are readily available. This is not the case in many areas of the world, and in general only areas where water is available have become populated. Even where it is available, it may be, or become, contaminated with toxins or infectious agents and become a major threat to health. One of the earliest tasks in dealing with any major disaster is to restore or supply safe drinking water.

HOMEOSTASIS

Water homeostasis requires that intake is sufficient to match total output (and, in children, the requirements of growth). Renal output is relatively easy to measure; faecal output is less so, and losses in sweat and the expired gas usually have to be estimated.

Homeostasis is achieved through the hypothalamus, where osmoreceptors sense plasma osmolality and respond by affecting the sensation of thirst and controlling the release of vasopressin (antidiuretic hormone) from the posterior pituitary gland. In the kidneys, the countercurrent system allows the production of dilute or concentrated urine in response to the concentration of vasopressin in the blood. An increase in plasma osmolality induces a sensation of thirst and stimulates the release of vasopressin. This stimulates the insertion of aquaporins (water channels) into the luminal membranes of cells in the renal collecting ducts, which are otherwise impermeable to water. This allows the passive movement of water into the interstitium down the concentration gradient generated by the countercurrent system and concentrates the urine. If plasma osmolality falls, the sensation of thirst is quenched, vasopressin secretion is minimised and the kidneys produce dilute urine.

This mechanism is exquisitely sensitive and, in health, ensures that plasma osmolality is maintained in the range 285-295 mmol/kg. Many other factors can also influence thirst and vasopressin secretion, notably hypovolaemia (which stimulates both), but these are more important pathologically than physiologically. In water deprivation, the effect on extracellular fluid volume is ameliorated by a shift of water from the much larger intracellular compartment, and *vice versa*, but in either case this apparently protective mechanism can lead to potentially dangerous consequences (e.g. cerebral oedema in acute water overload).

Despite the undoubted physiological importance of thirst as a stimulus to drink, for most free-living individuals in developed countries, fluid intake is determined by habit and by social factors. Unconsciousness, confusion, being unable to respond to thirst because of age, disability or physical restraint are all threats to adequate hydration. So, too, are the very rare conditions in which the function of the thirst centre is impaired.

DEFICIENCY
Thirst is the earliest effect of water deficiency, being stimulated by the inevitable increase in plasma osmolality as the decrease in water leads to increased concentration of solutes. There is decreased secretion of mucus and saliva, leading to a dry mouth and difficulty with swallowing. Urine volume falls (except when excessive renal loss is the cause) and the urine becomes highly concentrated (osmolality >1000 mmol/kg). There is hypernatraemia and haemoconcentration. Dehydration causes lethargy and physical weakness, followed in severe cases by confusion, coma and, without treatment, death (Figure 2.1). The term 'dehydration' is often applied loosely to the clinical state arising from the loss of any fluid from the body. It should be appreciated that the loss of water (or hypotonic fluid) from the body is potentially less harmful than the loss of isotonic fluid. The loss

of the latter is borne primarily only by the extracellular compartment (including the plasma) in the short term, whereas the loss of hypotonic fluid is borne by the whole body water pool. This is illustrated in Figure 2.2.

EXCESS

Healthy kidneys have a considerable capacity to excrete water (up to 30 L/24 h for short periods) so that water excess is very rare in healthy individuals. It can, however, occur with massive fluid intake (e.g. psychogenic polydipsia), especially if the solute content of the fluid is low, or with the absorption of hypotonic irrigation fluid during prostatic surgery. Water excess may also occur if water excretion is impaired, e.g. in renal failure, or when diuresis is compromised by an increase in vasopressin secretion, such as can occur acutely following trauma or chronically in the syndrome of inappropriate antidiuresis. The reader requiring more information on these topics should consult a textbook of clinical biochemistry. Hyponatraemia is invariably present. The clinical effects of water overload are primarily the result of an osmotically driven movement of water into the cells of the central nervous system, and are summarised in Figure 2.1. In general, acute water excess is more likely to be symptomatic than chronic water excess.

Features of water depletion and excess

	Water depletion	Water excess
Clinical features	Thirst	Confusion
	Dryness of mouth	Headache
	Difficulty swallowing	Convulsions
	Oliguria (early)	Coma
	Weakness	Extensor plantar reflexes
	Confusion	Weight gain
	Coma	
Laboratory features	Hypernatraemia	Hyponatraemia
	Haemoconcentration	Haemodilution
	Concentrated urine	

Figure 2.1 Features of water depletion and excess

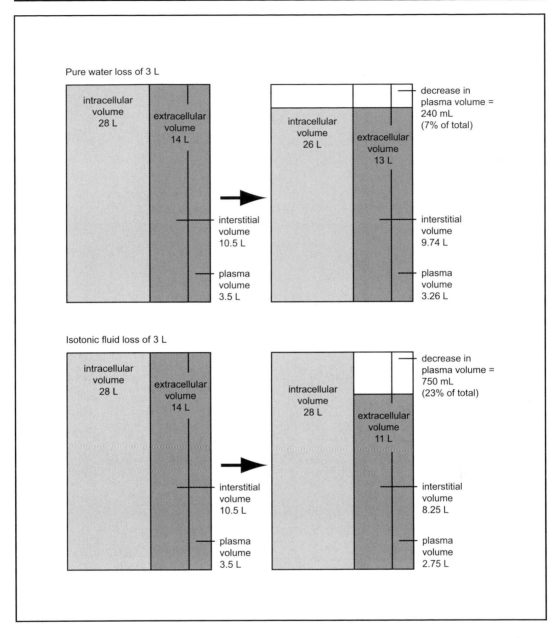

Figure 2.2 The comparative effects of the loss of equal volumes of isotonic fluid or water from the extracellular fluid. Loss of isotonic fluid has a greater effect on plasma volume because loss of water leads to an osmotic gradient, which results in a compensatory movement of water from the extracellular to the intracellular fluid so that the loss is borne by the whole water pool.

ASSESSMENT OF STATUS

This requires both clinical assessment and laboratory investigations, particularly of plasma sodium concentration (or osmolality). It should be noted that while in general plasma osmolality is primarily determined by the water content of the extracellular fluid, it can be increased by a high concentration of solute, e.g. sodium or glucose. In the short term, changes in body weight are a reliable guide to changes in hydration.

It is beyond the scope of this book to discuss the management of water depletion and overload in detail. The general principles are to treat the underlying cause, where possible. Water overload should usually be treated by restriction of intake but occasionally, in water intoxication, more active measures are required. Water depletion should be treated by giving water orally or 5% dextrose intravenously. In both conditions, it is important not to attempt to normalise plasma osmolality too rapidly, particularly if the disorder is chronic.

Carbohydrates

FUNCTION

Carbohydrates of nutritional value include poly-, oligo- and monosaccharides. The most abundant polysaccharide is starch, a polymer of glucose with α1-6 linkages. Disaccharides include maltose (two glucose residues), sucrose (glucose and fructose) and lactose (glucose and galactose). Though no carbohydrate has been shown to be an essential nutrient *per se*, they are collectively the major source of energy in most diets (exceptions include the Inuit races, whose major natural source of energy is fat). Carbohydrates provide 4 kcal energy (16.7 kJoules) per gram.

SOURCES

Digestible polysaccharides are present in numerous vegetable products, including grains, pulses and fruit, and are a major component of the staple food (e.g. rice, maize, cassava) in many areas of the world. Refined sugars (primarily sucrose) are widely available and are ubiquitous in processed foods, carbonated drinks, biscuits, confectionery and many other products.

HOMEOSTASIS

Energy homeostasis is achieved through a complex interaction of neural and hormonal mechanisms and is exquisitely sensitive to the body's requirements. An average healthy adult male may consume food with an energy content of approximately 9×10^5 kcals (3.76×10^6 kJoules) in a year, equivalent to about 130 kg non-aqueous body mass, yet without a significant increase or decrease in body weight.

DEFICIENCY

Starvation frequently involves a lack of adequate dietary carbohydrates but, because no carbohydrate is individually essential for health, there is no specific syndrome associated with carbohydrate deficiency alone.

EXCESS

An excessive intake of carbohydrates, i.e. that supplies more than the body's energy requirements, leads to obesity (see Chapter 6) and is an important factor in the pathogenesis of insulin resistance and hence type 2 diabetes mellitus.

ASSESSMENT OF STATUS

Only the liver and muscle can store significant quantities of carbohydrate, in the form of glycogen. Glucose derived from muscle glycogen is only available to that tissue: glucose derived from hepatic glycogen is secreted into the blood. Hepatic glycogen stores become depleted within 18-24 h if no carbohydrate is ingested, whereafter blood glucose is maintained by gluconeogenesis from amino acids, lactate and glycerol.

Blood glucose concentration thus does not provide an indication of the body's carbohydrate reserves. Dietary carbohydrate in excess of immediate requirements is converted into fat. The assessment of fat stores – the body's major energy store – is discussed in Chapter 4.

DIETARY FIBRE

All foods of vegetable origin contain complex carbohydrates that cannot be digested in the small intestine. These fibres (sometimes referred to as non-starch polysaccharides, NSP) include celluloses, hemicelluloses, pectins, gums and mucilages. The latter three are water-soluble. Lignins are also fibres, but are non-carbohydrate, being polymers of aromatic alcohols. The water-soluble NSP undergo metabolism by colonic bacteria, producing short-chain fatty acids (e.g. propionic acid), which can be absorbed, as well as carbon dioxide, hydrogen and methane.

The effects of dietary fibre have been extensively studied since it was first demonstrated that rural Africans, whose diet is high in fibre, have a low incidence of certain diseases, including bowel cancer. Dietary fibre increases stool bulk and is of value in the prevention of constipation. Major multinational trials have clearly demonstrated an association between a diet high in fibre and reduced risk of colonic adenomas and carcinomas. It has also been shown that soluble fibres will slow the rate of absorption of monosaccharides in the small intestine, which is of benefit in diabetes, and reduce total and LDL (low density lipoprotein) cholesterol concentrations without affecting HDL (high density lipoprotein) cholesterol. For all these reasons, it is considered that a healthy diet should contain approximately 30 g/day of non-starch polysaccharides.

Fats

FUNCTION

The major dietary fat is triglycerides (strictly, triacylglycerols). In triglycerides of animal origin, the component fatty acid residues are in the main saturated; in those derived from vegetables and fish, the fatty acids are for the most part unsaturated. The major function of dietary triglycerides is as a source of energy (approximately 9 kcal/g (37.6 kJoules/g)). Dietary fat also includes cholesterol and other sterols, phospholipids and the fat soluble vitamins (A, D, E and K).

The major saturated fatty acids in the body are palmitic acid (C16), stearic (C18) and myristic (C14) acids. The number refers to the total number of carbon atoms. In unsaturated fatty acids, the figure following this number indicates the number of double bonds: their positions (from the terminal methyl group) are given by the figure(s) following the letter ω (Greek omega) (see Figure 2.3). The preferred scientific nomenclature is similar but ω is replaced by Δ, and the following numbers indicate the position of the double bonds starting from the carboxy end of the molecule. The number of carbon atoms is also indicated by the systematic name: thus linoleic acid is C18:2, ω6,9 or C18:2 $\Delta^{9,12}$, that is, $\Delta^{9,12}$ octadecadienoic acid.

The chemical structure of linoleic, α-linolenic and arachidonic acids

$CH_3(CH_2)_4CH=CHCH_2CH=CH(CH_2)_7COOH$
Linoleic ($\Delta^{9,12}$ octadecadienoic) acid (C18:2)

$CH_3CH_2CH=CHCH_2CH=CHCH_2CH=CH(CH_2)_7COOH$
α-Linolenic ($\Delta^{9,12,15}$ octadecatrienoic) acid (C18:3)

$CH_3(CH_2)_4CH=CHCH_2CH=CHCH_2CH=CHCH_2CH=CH(CH_2)_3COOH$
Arachidonic ($\Delta^{5,8,11,14}$ eicosatetraenoic) acid (C20:4)

Figure 2.3 The chemical structure of linoleic, α-linolenic and arachidonic acids. The systematic names are given in brackets. The double bonds are in the *cis* configuration

Small amounts of two unsaturated fatty acids (linolenic acid (C18:3, ω3,6,9) and linoleic acid) are essential: they are precursors of prostanoids, such as prostacyclins and thromboxanes. Arachidonic acid (C20:4, ω6,9,12,15) is also involved in prostanoid synthesis but although it cannot be synthesised *de novo* it can be produced from linoleic acid. Other functions of essential fatty acids include maintenance of the epidermal barrier to water in the skin (particularly linoleic acid), maintenance of normal immune function and growth and, in the case of omega-3 acids, a structural role in cell membranes. Their effects on growth and immune function may be in part related to their role in cell membranes.

Unsaturated fatty acids can exist in *cis* or *trans* forms. Those that occur naturally are in the *cis* form, but the hydrogenation of vegetable oils (high in unsaturates) to increase the proportion of saturates (a process employed in the manufacture of margarine) leads to the production of *trans* unsaturated fatty acids. These cannot act as essential fatty acids and may interfere with the metabolism of naturally occurring unsaturated fatty acids. They tend to increase LDL cholesterol and reduce HDL cholesterol concentrations in the plasma and thus can be considered indirectly atherogenic. In this respect they resemble saturated fatty acids.

There is considerable evidence that a diet high in saturated fats predisposes to cardiovascular and other diseases. In contrast, epidemiological studies have demonstrated an association between a high intake of omega-3 *cis* unsaturated fatty acids and a reduced risk of cardiovascular disease. Supplementation of the diet with omega-3 *cis* unsaturated fatty acids has been demonstrated to increase plasma HDL cholesterol concentrations, to stabilise atheromatous plaques and to have a beneficial effect in the secondary prevention of cardiovascular disease. Although omega-6 *cis* unsaturated fatty acids tend to lower LDL cholesterol concentrations, there is evidence that a high ratio of omega-6 to omega-3 fats in the diet may adversely affect cardiovascular risk, and that this can be reduced by increasing the proportion of omega-3 unsaturated fats in the diet.

Current recommendations for dietary fat intake in the UK are that:

- energy intake as fat should be no more than 35% (ideally only 30%) of total requirements (in practice achieving less than 35% is difficult)

- no more than one third of this should be supplied by saturated fats

- *cis*-monounsaturated fatty acids should supply about 12% of dietary energy requirements, with the rest supplied by omega-3 and omega-6 polyunsaturated fatty acids in a ratio of 1:3-4.

SOURCES

All meat from animals contains triglycerides although in general the amounts are less in many wild animals (e.g. deer) than in domesticated beasts. Even lean meat contains some fat. In the vegetable kingdom, fats are found predominantly in fruits and seeds, e.g. nuts, olives, sunflower seeds and avocados, and are present in only small amounts in grains and pulses. Some vegetable sources contain primarily saturated fat (e.g. coconut); others are rich in mono- and/or polyunsaturated fatty acids. The unsaturated fats in most vegetables are primarily omega-6. 'Oily' fish, e.g. salmon and mackerel, are a rich source of polyunsaturated fats (particularly omega-3) although to some extent the fatty acids present in fish, in common with mammals, reflect their fat intake.

HOMEOSTASIS

Energy homeostasis is discussed briefly in Chapter 6. It is beyond the scope of this book to discuss in detail the complex interactions between the metabolism of triglycerides and carbohydrates that ensure that energy in excess of the body's immediate requirements is stored and made available during fasting. It may be noted, however, that the body's stores of triglycerides are considerable. Even in a lean adult male, they may constitute 15 kg, equivalent to 136 Mcals (570 MJoules), or 54 days' normal energy expenditure.

DEFICIENCY

Apart from the essential fatty acids, triglycerides are not an essential component of the diet. In areas of the world where there is a high prevalence of starvation, fat is normally only a minor component of the diet. In developed countries, a poor energy intake usually involves an inadequate intake of both carbohydrate and fat. Adults store considerable quantities of essential fatty acids and isolated clinical deficiency is rare, although it has been described in patients on total parenteral nutrition with restricted fat content. Infants have low stores, and are more susceptible to deficiency, especially if premature. The earliest clinical feature of deficiency of essential fatty acids is dermatitis, which can lead to increased water loss. Impaired function of cell membranes leads to increased capillary permeability and fragility of red blood cells. With severe deficiency, growth may be adversely affected. Impaired learning ability has been demonstrated in experimental animals with essential fatty acid deficiency.

EXCESS

Many conditions, including obesity, cardiovascular disease and some cancers, are associated with a high dietary fat intake. In developed countries, however, despite the existence of recommendations to reduce fat intake, many individuals consume excessive amounts of fat, not helped by the high fat content and ready availability of many 'fast foods', snacks and other semi-manufactured foods.

ASSESSMENT OF STATUS

The body's stores of fat can be measured using various physical and anthropometric measurements (see Chapter 4). Fasting plasma triglyceride concentrations tend to be increased in individuals in whom body fat is increased, but the relationship is neither sufficiently sensitive nor specific for their measurement to be of value in assessing fat stores.

In essential fatty acid deficiency, increased desaturation and elongation of oleic acid leads to the formation of Mead acid (C20:3 ω9,12,15). Essential fatty acid status can be assessed by measuring the ratio of Mead acid to linoleic acid in plasma membrane lipids: this is normally <0.1; a ratio >0.4 is indicative of deficiency.

Proteins

FUNCTION

Proteins are polymers of amino acids. Over 20 amino acids occur in the human body, of which eight are essential. These are isoleucine, leucine, lysine, methionine, phenylalanine, threonine, tryptophan and valine. Histidine is an essential amino acid for infants. The other amino acids can all be synthesised in the body. However, a limited intake of certain amino acids may impose an absolute requirement for others that are produced from them: an example is tyrosine, which can be synthesised from phenylalanine, and must be supplemented in people with phenylketonuria, who are treated with phenylalanine restriction. Dietary protein is required both as a source of the essential amino acids and as a source of nitrogen, for the synthesis of proteins, purines, pyrimidines and other nitrogen-containing substances.

Although most amino acids or their nitrogen can be reutilised in the body, there is a constant obligatory loss of nitrogen from the body, mostly in the urine, and to a lesser extent in faeces and desquamated skin. Assuming adequate energy provision as carbohydrate and fat (to minimise the requirement for protein to be sacrificed for gluconeogenesis) and an adequate content of essential amino acids, the recommended dietary intake of protein for adults is ~0.75 g/kg body weight per day, equivalent to ~4.5 mmol elemental nitrogen. A greater intake may be required to provide adequate quantities of essential amino acids if the protein is relatively deficient in any of these; in general, vegetable proteins are inferior to animal proteins in this respect. Nitrogen requirements in children are greater because of the demands of growth. Requirements in adults can be increased under several circumstances, for example, during recovery from illness, when catabolised protein is being replaced.

The carbon skeletons of many amino acids can become a source of glucose; others are ketogenic. The nitrogen made available during gluconeogenesis and amino acid oxidation is excreted mainly as urea in urine; increased protein turnover (e.g. in a catabolic state) and a high dietary protein intake will increase urea production and hence the load on the kidneys.

It should be noted that the body is only able to utilise L-amino acids; naturally occurring proteins only contain L-amino acids, but chemical synthesis produces racemic mixtures, and this must be taken into account in the preparation of amino acid mixtures used in parenteral nutrition support.

SOURCES

All unrefined animal and vegetable matter contains protein, but there are considerable quantitative and qualitative differences. In general, meat and fish are richer in protein than vegetables, and the quality of protein (i.e. its content of essential amino acids) is greater in meat and fish than vegetables. The protein content of pulses is higher than that of green vegetables.

HOMEOSTASIS

It is beyond the scope of this book to discuss the complex regulation of amino acid and protein metabolism in the body. Rates of protein synthesis and breakdown are controlled by the endocrine system; when dietary protein intake is low changes may occur to ameliorate the potential effects of the decreased availability of amino acids for protein synthesis. For example, in simple starvation (i.e. not accompanied by sepsis or another cause of increased catabolism), the fractional catabolic rate of albumin falls, so that its half life in the plasma is increased. It should be remembered, however, that if energy intake is also less than requirements, there will be an increased obligatory requirement for amino acids to be diverted to gluconeogenesis to provide energy, rather than to protein synthesis.

DEFICIENCY

The consequences of protein deficiency depend to some extent on whether this is an isolated phenomenon, or an aspect of overall malnutrition. In children, lack of sufficient energy substrates and proteins leads to generalised wasting, or marasmus (see Chapter 1) whereas lack of protein alone leads to kwashiorkor. In both conditions, however, and in the intermediate forms of protein malnutrition, there is gradual loss both of structural proteins and of plasma and other proteins. The former leads to muscle weakness and decreased mobility, the latter to various functional defects including increased susceptibility to infection as a result of decreased synthesis of immunoglobulins and impaired wound healing. Growth slows or, in severe cases, ceases altogether.

Similar features occur in adults with dietary protein deficiency (except the lack of growth), but kwashiorkor does not appear to develop in adults on a protein deficient but energy replete diet. If protein intake is inadequate, deficiencies of other nutrients are also likely and may impinge significantly on the clinical presentation.

EXCESS

There is little evidence that a high protein diet is directly of potential harm in healthy individuals, although the expense of protein renders this an unlikely problem for the majority of the world's population. Some supposedly therapeutic diets (e.g. Atkins) recommend a high protein intake. Nitrogen surplus to the body's requirements is converted mainly to urea and excreted in the urine; the obligatory osmotic load for the kidneys and hence obligatory water excretion will be increased in consequence. Plasma urea concentrations tend to be higher in individuals with normal renal function consuming large amounts of protein, but there is no evidence that this is harmful and renal function itself is not compromised. However, the fact that a high protein intake almost invariably means a high purine intake is potentially harmful, and may lead to hyperuricaemia, an increased risk of gout in susceptible individuals and an increased risk of urate-containing urinary calculi.

Avoidance of an unnecessarily high protein intake is important for two groups of patients: those with renal disease and those with chronic liver disease. A high protein intake increases the burden on failing kidneys and there is evidence that the rate of progression of chronic renal disease may be slowed by reducing protein intake (albeit not to an extent that leads to negative nitrogen balance). Limitation of protein intake is also of proven benefit to reduce the risk of encephalopathy in patients with chronic liver disease; again, it should not be so severe as to cause negative nitrogen balance.

ASSESSMENT OF STATUS

Many techniques have been described for assessing protein status. These include estimation of overall nitrogen balance, indirect assessment of skeletal muscle mass, functional measurements of muscle strength and measurements of individual plasma proteins. The relative merits of these are discussed in Chapter 4.

Major inorganic nutrients

Calcium

FUNCTION

Calcium is a major component of hydroxyapatite, the predominant mineral in bone and teeth (which together contain 99% of the body's calcium), but calcium is essential to many fundamental processes in the body, including blood coagulation, muscle contraction, neuromuscular transmission, the control of transmembrane ion channels and intracellular signalling. Intracellular calcium concentrations (approximately 0.1 μmol/L) are very low in relation to those of plasma (which are some 20,000 times higher) and are kept low by a combination of the actions of an ATPase dependent calcium pump and exchange for sodium. Small increases in intracellular calcium concentration are responsible for many processes, such as the secretion of hormones in response to the binding of effectors to membrane receptors. Complex mechanisms exist for regulating the concentration of calcium in the extracellular fluid and the fluxes of calcium between various organs. Dietary calcium is incompletely absorbed from the gut and this, together with active secretion, results in significant obligatory faecal loss of calcium. The recommended calcium intake for adults is about 800 mg (20 mmol) per day (higher in the USA than the UK); much higher intakes are required during childhood, pregnancy and lactation.

SOURCES

Milk and dairy products are the richest dietary sources of calcium; pulses and leafy vegetables contain calcium but in some vegetables, e.g. spinach, the presence of oxalic acid limits its bioavailability. Fish that are consumed whole, such as whitebait and sardines, are also rich sources. The absorption of dietary calcium is controlled by calcitriol but is affected by numerous dietary constituents: oxalate, phytates, phosphate and free fatty acids all combine with calcium ions and can reduce absorption.

HOMEOSTASIS

Calcium homeostasis is complex. Two principal hormones are involved: parathyroid hormone (PTH), a peptide hormone secreted by the parathyroids, and calcitriol (1,25-dihydroxycholecalciferol), the hormone derived from vitamin D (p.69). These hormones act synergistically. The major function of calcitriol is to increase the absorption of dietary calcium from the gut, whereas shorter term regulation of plasma calcium concentration is effected largely by PTH, which stimulates calcium resorption from bone (an action in part dependent on calcitriol), calcium reabsorption in the kidneys and the activation of vitamin D. A third hormone, calcitonin, can be demonstrated to inhibit osteoclastic activity but appears to have only a minor role in calcium homeostasis. States of calcitonin deficiency or excess are not associated with abnormal calcium homeostasis.

DEFICIENCY AND EXCESS

Because most of the calcium in the body is present in the skeleton, whereas the homeostatic mechanisms act primarily to maintain the plasma calcium concentration in the physiological range, hypo- and hypercalcaemia do not necessarily reflect calcium deficiency or excess. Furthermore, the homeostatic mechanisms can defend plasma calcium concentration by increasing the resorption of bone mineral. Disorders of calcium concentration usually reflect disorders of its hormonal control, e.g. hypo- and hyperparathyroidism or deficiency/excess of vitamin D. The most obvious feature of hypocalcaemia is increased neuromuscular excitability, leading to muscle spasm, tetany and even convulsions. The effects of hypercalcaemia are less specific, and include polyuria, abdominal pain, anorexia, changes in mentation and, if chronic, an increased risk of renal calculus formation.

Calcium deficiency in childhood and adolescence may contribute to an increased risk of osteoporosis in later life. Bone mass depends on the peak bone mass attained (typically at age 20-25 years) and the rate of later net bone loss. An adequate calcium intake is one of the determinants of peak bone mass. However, osteoporosis has a multifactorial pathogenesis, with potentially both decreased bone formation and increased bone breakdown being involved. Bone is continually undergoing remodelling as a result of the activity of osteoclasts (cells that break down bone) and osteoblasts (cells involved in bone formation). Remodelling is normally a coordinated process, controlled largely by paracrine factors, and any disruption of this control can lead to overall loss of bone mineral.

ASSESSMENT OF STATUS

Plasma calcium is easily measured in the laboratory. About half the calcium in the blood is present as free calcium ions and is biologically active; the rest is mainly complexed with albumin, with a small amount combined with phosphate. Since total calcium concentration is in part dependent on the concentration of albumin in the plasma, many laboratories report a 'corrected calcium' – in essence, an estimate, in patients with abnormal albumin concentrations, of what the calcium would be if the albumin concentration were normal. Ionised calcium can be measured directly, but is best suited to point of care instruments as it can change rapidly in blood *in vitro*.

The diagnosis of osteoporosis is based on measurements of bone mineral density, which reflect total body calcium. Bone mineral density is most accurately measured by dual X-ray absorptiometry (DEXA).

Chlorine

FUNCTION AND SOURCES

Chloride is the principal extracellular anion. It is thus important, together with sodium, in the maintenance of extracellular fluid volume, but does not appear to have a role independently of sodium. It is secreted together with hydrogen ions into the lumen of the stomach: the role of gastric acid is discussed in Chapter 3. Chlorine is widely available in foods as the chlorides of sodium and potassium.

DEFICIENCY AND EXCESS

Chloride deficiency and excess usually accompany deficiency and excess of sodium. However, two specific chloride-losing states are of interest: loss of chloride as hydrochloric acid from the stomach in patients having gastric fluid aspirated or with vomiting secondary to pyloric stenosis, and chloride-losing diarrhoea, a rare condition that can occur as a congenital disorder in infants or be a complication of cystic fibrosis. The specific effect of chloride loss is metabolic alkalosis, in part caused by a combination of increased renal bicarbonate absorption, and by increased aldosterone secretion and potassium deficiency, both of which promote increased renal hydrogen ion excretion. It is treated by the intravenous administration of isotonic (0.9%) saline. This type of hypochloraemic alkalosis, in which there is an element of hypovolaemia, is termed saline- (or chloride-) responsive metabolic alkalosis. In contrast, hypochloraemic alkalosis secondary to hyperaldosteronism or potassium depletion is not accompanied by volume depletion and is termed saline- (or chloride-) resistant alkalosis.

The administration of inappropriately large volumes of isotonic (0.9%) sodium chloride solution can lead to acidosis ('dilution acidosis'). The chloride concentration of the infused fluid is greater than that of the plasma but that of sodium is about the same. Thus plasma sodium concentration remains normal but there is a tendency for chloride concentration to rise and the maintenance of electrochemical neutrality results in a fall in bicarbonate concentration. This is the reverse of the 'contraction alkalosis' that can sometimes occur in patients with oedema given high doses of diuretics.

ASSESSMENT OF STATUS

Plasma chloride concentration reflects both the amount of chloride in the extracellular fluid and the amount of water (see sodium, p.41); changes in chloride concentration usually parallel changes in sodium concentration, except in hypochloraemic alkalosis (see above) and hyperchloraemic acidosis (e.g. renal tubular acidosis). Measurements of urine chloride excretion may help to distinguish between chloride-responsive alkalosis (urine chloride <10 mmol/L) and chloride-resistant alkalosis (urine chloride typically greater than 10 mmol/L).

Magnesium

FUNCTION

Magnesium is the fourth most abundant cation in the body. Only 1% of the total is in the extracellular fluid, where its concentration is approximately 1 mmol/L, about half of which is free magnesium ions. Approximately two thirds is found in bone and one third in cells, mainly muscle. Magnesium ions are a cofactor for numerous reactions in the body, particularly those involving ATP and protein synthesis.

SOURCES AND HOMEOSTASIS

Magnesium is widely distributed in foodstuffs, with green vegetables being a particularly rich source (magnesium is a component of chlorophyll). Dietary magnesium intake is approximately 15 mmol/day (360 mg/day), of which about one third is absorbed, although the proportion that is absorbed is regulated in relation to the body's requirements. Control is effected primarily through the amount of magnesium excreted in the urine; fractional magnesium reabsorption from the tubular fluid increases in magnesium depletion. Unusually in comparison with other ions, the major site of magnesium reabsorption is the thick ascending limb of the loop of Henle.

DEFICIENCY

Isolated magnesium deficiency is uncommon: it is usually associated with other fluid and electrolyte disturbances. Magnesium depletion can occur as a result of dietary insufficiency or decreased absorption, increased loss from the gut (e.g. in severe diarrhoea or ileostomy fluid) and increased renal loss (as can be induced by loop and thiazide diuretics, and by other drugs, such as amphotericin, aminoglycosides, cisplatin and ciclosporin). Excessive gastrointestinal loss of sodium and water (e.g. in patients with an ileostomy) can cause secondary hyperaldosteronism, which also stimulates renal magnesium loss and exacerbates magnesium depletion. Hypomagnesaemia without magnesium depletion can occur in acute pancreatitis, owing to the formation of insoluble magnesium salts with fatty acids (as can occur with calcium). The early features of hypomagnesaemia are non-specific (e.g. nausea, apathy, depression) but severe or prolonged hypomagnesaemia can cause potassium depletion (as a result of decreased activity of Na^+,K^+-ATPase) and hypocalcaemia (parathyroid hormone secretion is magnesium dependent). Severe hypomagnesaemia is associated with cardiac dysrhythmias and neuromuscular symptoms (muscle weakness, twitching and tetany): these are believed to be consequences of hypokalaemia and hypocalcaemia, respectively, rather than direct effects of magnesium depletion.

Management should be directed at the underlying cause, and magnesium can be replaced by slow intravenous infusion (up to 50 mmol/24 h) when necessary.

Two inherited disorders can cause magnesium depletion. Isolated dominant hypomagnesaemia is due to a mutation of the *FXYD2* gene, which encodes part of a renal Na^+,K^+-ATPase. Decreased activity leads to a decrease in potassium entry into tubular cells, which reduces potassium-dependent magnesium reabsorption. In familial hypomagnesaemia, hypercalciuria and nephrocalcinosis (FHHNC), there is defective renal reabsorption of magnesium and calcium, often associated with other tubular abnormalities; the nephrocalcinosis leads to progressive renal failure. This condition is caused by mutations in the *CLND16* gene, which codes for a protein involved in the formation of tight junctions.

EXCESS

Control of intestinal absorption and renal excretion ensures that a high magnesium intake does not lead to hypermagnesaemia in patients with normal renal function. It is usually seen in patients with renal failure, and occasionally in patients taking magnesium-containing purgatives or antacids. Clinical features typically only occur with concentrations greater than 2 mmol/L: they are related to decreased neuromuscular excitability, e.g. hyporeflexia, respiratory paralysis and cardiac conduction defects. High magnesium concentrations are directly toxic, inhibiting acetylcholine release. Magnesium is used therapeutically to control the seizures of eclampsia (pregnancy-associated hypertension).

The management of hypermagnesaemia should be directed to the underlying cause, which usually requires renal replacement therapy. In the short term, intravenous calcium, with dextrose and insulin, is an effective magnesium antagonist.

ASSESSMENT OF STATUS

Plasma magnesium concentration is easily measured. A magnesium loading test, in which renal excretion following a parenteral load is measured, can be used to assess total body magnesium but is rarely required in clinical practice. Erythrocyte magnesium concentrations have been studied as an index of total body magnesium status. Although low concentrations are typical of depletion, the reference interval is wide and erythrocyte magnesium concentration tends to fall as cells age, from an initial level determined by magnesium status at the time of erythropoiesis.

Phosphorus

FUNCTION AND SOURCES

Phosphorus has numerous functions in the body, being a component of high energy phosphates, nucleic acids, intracellular signalling molecules and bone, and having a critical role in metabolic control through changes in the activity of enzymes depending on whether they are phosphorylated or dephosphorylated. Not surprisingly, phosphorus is present in all natural foods. Dietary deficiency has not been described, except in starvation.

HOMEOSTASIS

The control of plasma phosphate concentration is closely linked to that of calcium. Parathyroid hormone liberates calcium and phosphate from bone but is phosphaturic, hence patients with hyperparathyroidism are typically hypophosphataemic and hypoparathyroidism can cause hyperphosphataemia. Calcitriol increases the absorption of dietary phosphate.

DEFICIENCY AND HYPOPHOSPHATAEMIA

Although dietary deficiency does not occur, the absorption of phosphate from the gut can be decreased by the ingestion of aluminium hydroxide, which binds to it. Indeed, this salt, sometimes used as an antacid, has in the past been used therapeutically to limit phosphate absorption in patients with renal failure.

Hypophosphataemia can be a consequence of inadequate intake, increased gut or renal losses, or redistribution (e.g. increased cellular uptake). The many causes include inadequate parenteral provision, the refeeding syndrome (see p.151), 'hungry bone disease' (sometimes seen after parathyroidectomy) and alcohol withdrawal.

Mild hypophosphataemia is clinically inconsequential, but concentrations of less than 0.4 mmol/L can lead to muscle weakness (including diaphragmatic weakness, which may cause problems with respiration or weaning patients off ventilators), impaired delivery of oxygen to tissues (due to reduced red cell 2,3-bisphosphoglycerate concentrations leading to a left shift in the oxygen-haemoglobin dissociation curve) and impaired white cell function. If hypophosphataemia requires urgent treatment, sodium or potassium phosphate should be given intravenously at a rate of not more than 9 mmol/12 h, with frequent monitoring of plasma calcium and phosphate concentrations: over-rapid provision can cause severe hypocalcaemia.

EXCESS AND HYPERPHOSPHATAEMIA

In the past, a high phosphate intake as a result of feeding undiluted cows' milk to infants was a well-recognised cause of hyperphosphataemia, but in general, except in renal failure, a high dietary intake is not harmful. Phosphate used to be given intravenously to treat severe hypercalcaemia, but this is no longer recommended because of the risk of metastatic calcification. The major cause of hyperphosphataemia now is renal failure, and the main problem associated with it is its tendency to combine with calcium and precipitate in blood vessels, periarticular structures and other tissues. Oral phosphate binders are used to reduce its severity.

INHERITED DISORDERS AFFECTING PLASMA PHOSPHATE CONCENTRATION
Chronic hypophosphataemia can cause defective bone mineralisation, and this is a feature of several rare, inherited disorders in which there is reduced renal tubular reabsorption of phosphate. They include X-linked and autosomal dominant hypophosphataemic rickets, in which mutations cause impaired degradation of phosphatonins (e.g. fibroblast growth factor 23), resulting in inhibition of the proximal renal sodium-phosphate cotransporter, and Dent's disease, a group of hereditary tubular disorders in which there is a defect in a proximal tubular endosomal chloride channel that results in locally increased PTH-related effects, possibly owing to reduced renal degradation of parathyroid hormone.

ASSESSMENT OF STATUS
The plasma concentration of phosphate is easily measured. It may occasionally be necessary to assess the ability of the kidneys to reabsorb filtered phosphate (TmP/GFR) in the investigation of chronic hypophosphataemia, but measuring 24 h phosphate excretion is of no clinical value.

Potassium

FUNCTION
Potassium is the principal intracellular anion: the concentration in the intracellular fluid is approximately 120 mmol/L, and in the extracellular fluid, 4.0 mmol/L. Potassium can freely diffuse out of cells so maintenance of this large concentration gradient (and the gradient of sodium concentration in the opposite direction) is an energy dependent process driven by a Na^+,K^+-ATPase (the Na^+,K^+-pump). The difference between the concentrations of potassium across cell membranes is the principal determinant of the resting membrane potential that governs the excitability of nerve and muscle cells. The major clinical manifestations of disorders of potassium homeostasis are due to its effects on the membrane potential.

Because the bulk of the body's 3500 mmol of potassium (adult male) is intracellular, the plasma concentration may not reflect total body potassium. Although hypokalaemia usually signifies potassium depletion, this is not always the case, and hyperkalaemia can occur without there being an excess.

SOURCES
Potassium is widely distributed in foods of animal and vegetable origin. Dietary deficiency is unusual except during starvation, though potassium depletion may occur with an apparently adequate intake if there are excessive losses. Most people consume well in excess of the minimal requirement (40-60 mmol/day, or 1.5-2.3 g/day, assuming normal losses).

HOMEOSTASIS
Maintenance of normal body potassium content is dependent on the balance between intake and excretion; additionally, the maintenance of a normal plasma concentration depends on the distribution of potassium between the intra- and extracellular compartments. Because of the concentration difference, only a small perturbation of the mechanisms that normally maintain the gradient can have significant effects on extracellular concentration.

Potassium is readily absorbed, but also excreted, by the gut: approximately 10% of the amount excreted daily is lost in the stools. Increased gastrointestinal potassium loss can occur with vomiting and, particularly, with diarrhoea. In the kidneys, potassium is absorbed in the proximal convoluted tubules and secreted distally. Secretion is increased by aldosterone, production of which is stimulated by hyperkalaemia. Potassium depletion decreases aldosterone secretion. The secretion of potassium takes place in response to the reabsorption of sodium: hydrogen ions can replace potassium in this role, and in systemic alkalosis, potassium excretion is enhanced. However, since the major stimulus for the secretion of aldosterone is a decrease in extracellular fluid volume (sodium deficiency) the renal mechanisms for maintaining plasma potassium status are somewhat inefficient. In addition, the obligatory renal loss of potassium depends to some extent on the rate of urine formation, being higher at high urine flow rates.

Cellular uptake of potassium is stimulated by insulin and β-adrenergic drugs, and decreased in acidosis (when intracellular buffering of hydrogen ions leads to compensatory movement of potassium out of cells). Massive loss of intracellular potassium to the extracellular compartment occurs with damage to cell membranes, e.g. in trauma.

POTASSIUM DEPLETION AND HYPOKALAEMIA
Potassium depletion is usually a result of excess loss of potassium either from the gut or kidneys. The most common cause of persistent hypokalaemia is treatment with diuretics (thiazides and loop diuretics). Primary aldosteronism is an impor-

tant though less common cause: it also causes hypertension and should be considered in young people with hypertension and in patients with hypertension that is difficult to control with drugs. Hypokalaemia can also occur because of increased cellular uptake of potassium, for example during treatment with β-adrenergic agonists or insulin (e.g. in diabetic ketoacidosis). The surge in erythropoiesis following the treatment of pernicious anaemia with vitamin B_{12} can sometimes cause hypokalaemia for the same reason.

Mild hypokalaemia is usually asymptomatic, but severe hypokalaemia (i.e. <2.5 mmol/L) can cause muscle weakness. Cardiac arrhythmias may also occur. Hypokalaemia increases susceptibility to digoxin toxicity. Treatment should be directed to the underlying cause, with or without oral slow release potassium. If intravenous potassium is required, careful monitoring is essential to ensure that hyperkalaemia does not ensue, particularly in patients with renal insufficiency. An infusion rate of 20 mmol/h should be exceeded only with great caution.

POTASSIUM EXCESS AND HYPERKALAEMIA

The two major causes of potassium excess and hyperkalaemia are excessive therapeutic use of potassium and renal failure, both acute and chronic. Both potassium-sparing diuretics and angiotensin-converting enzyme (ACE) inhibitors can cause hyperkalaemia: they should be used with caution in patients with renal insufficiency. Their combined use is particularly hazardous. Loss of intracellular potassium to the extracellular compartment can cause hyperkalaemia without total body excess. This is the cause of the (self-limiting) hyperkalaemia that occurs after severe exercise. Loss of intracellular potassium *in vitro* (after a blood specimen has been obtained but before it is analysed) is a common problem; visible haemolysis is by no means always present.

Hyperkalaemia may give rise to no signs or symptoms until cardiac arrest occurs, usually in asystole. A potassium concentration of >7.0 mmol/L is a medical emergency; calcium chloride or gluconate (10 mL of 10% solution over 5 min) should be given intravenously to afford temporary protection to the myocardium; 50% dextrose (50 mL over 15 min) with 10 U soluble insulin drives potassium into cells. Both these can be repeated. In renal failure, renal replacement therapy (e.g. haemofiltration) may be required.

ASSESSMENT OF STATUS

Total body potassium can be measured using an isotope dilution technique. Plasma potassium concentration is important in its own right but may not be a good guide to total body potassium, although a concentration of <3.0 mmol/L usually implies a significant deficit. Measurement of urinary potassium is occasionally helpful to determine whether hypokalaemia is due to excessive renal loss.

With extrarenal losses, urinary potassium excretion is typically <25 mmol/L (provided that the patient is normally hydrated, as fluid depletion leads to increased secretion of aldosterone, which increases potassium excretion).

Sodium

FUNCTION

Sodium is the principal extracellular cation, being present at a concentration of approximately 140 mmol/L, while the intracellular concentration is 14 mmol/L; total body sodium is approximately 4000 mmol and half of this is in bone. Because of the sensitivity of the mechanisms controlling extracellular fluid osmolality (to which sodium makes a major contribution), the amount of sodium in the extra-cellular compartment is the major determinant of extracellular fluid volume.

Cell membranes are normally relatively impermeable to sodium. The concentra-tion gradient is maintained by the Na^+,K^+-pump. Depolarisation of the membranes of nerve and muscle cells is a result of the opening of sodium chan-nels and a rapid influx of sodium, causing the upstroke of the action potential.

The absorption of some nutrients from the gut is linked to the absorption of sodium – a fact made use of in the formulation of oral rehydration solutions, which contain both sodium and glucose.

SOURCES

Sodium is widely distributed in foods, though animal products generally contain more than vegetables. Salt is added to many manufactured foods both as a preser-vative and, supposedly, to enhance flavour. In addition, many people add salt to food during cooking or immediately prior to eating.

In a temperate climate, sodium balance can be maintained with an intake of less than 50 mmol/day (1.2 g/day or approximately 2.9 g/day sodium chloride). However, most people's intake is far higher than this. The relationship between salt intake and hypertension is discussed in Chapter 1.

HOMEOSTASIS

There are small obligatory losses of sodium in sweat and the faeces (though loss in sweat can be greatly increased with excessive sweating). Sodium balance is primarily maintained through the control of renal excretion. The factors that regu-late renal excretion include aldosterone, atrial natriuretic peptide, sympathetic activity and Starling forces in peritubular capillaries. Aldosterone is secreted as a result of activation of the renin-angiotensin-aldosterone axis in response to a decrease in renal perfusion, and stimulates distal renal sodium reabsorption.

Atrial natriuretic peptide, secreted in response to an increase in extracellular fluid volume, has various actions but in essence promotes sodium excretion by antagonising the actions of renin and through a direct effect on distal sodium reabsorption. Increased sympathetic nervous activity (prompted by a fall in blood pressure) causes vasoconstriction of afferent renal arterioles and promotes proximal sodium reabsorption. Expansion of the extracellular fluid volume tends to reduce the oncotic pressure, which decreases proximal renal tubular sodium reabsorption. It will be noted that these mechanisms relating to sodium homeostasis respond to changes in extracellular fluid volume or blood pressure because, as explained above, the sodium *content* of the extracellular fluid is the principal determinant of its *volume*.

DEFICIENCY
Sodium deficiency can arise as a result of a poor intake (unusual as a sole cause in healthy individuals) or because of increased losses through the skin, in the faeces or in the urine. A fall in plasma volume can also occur as a result of redistribution of extracellular fluid to the extravascular compartment, as occurs in oedema. Clinically important causes include loss of blood or plasma (e.g. burns), severe diarrhoea or vomiting and excessive use of diuretics. Peripheral vasodilation (e.g. in septic shock) can have similar consequences.

A fall in plasma volume leads to activation of sodium-conserving mechanisms, triggering increased renal sodium retention (provided that renal function and the other homeostatic mechanisms are intact) and, if severe, water retention through secretion of vasopressin. The clinical and laboratory features are summarised in Figure 2.4. Note that the plasma sodium concentration is not necessarily low. Sodium concentration depends both on the amounts of sodium and water, and mechanisms controlling osmolality tend to maintain osmolality (and hence sodium concentration) unless the deficit is severe. Note also that the clinical effects of loss of sodium (which must always be lost together with water) are more dangerous than the effects of the loss of similar volumes of water or hypotonic fluid: loss of isotonic fluid from the extracellular compartment does not cause an osmotic imbalance with respect to the intracellular fluid, so there is no compensatory movement of water as occurs with loss of hypotonic fluid (see Figure 2.2).

EXCESS
Sodium excess is usually iatrogenic. If homeostatic mechanisms are intact, it tends to cause expansion of the extracellular fluid volume, which leads to increased renal excretion primarily as a result of suppression of aldosterone secretion. There may be hypernatraemia, particularly with acute excess, but this is not invariable. The clinical and laboratory features of sodium excess are summarised in Figure 2.4.

Features of sodium deficiency and excess		
	Sodium deficiency	**Sodium excess**
Clinical features	Weakness	Peripheral oedema
	Apathy	Dyspnoea
	Postural dizziness	Pulmonary oedema
	Fainting	Effusions
	Tachycardia	Venous congestion
	Hypotension (initially postural)	Hypertension
	Cold peripheries (possibly cyanotic)	
	Decreased skin turgor	
	Decreased intraocular pressure	
	Oliguria (late)	
	Thirst (late)	
Laboratory features	Increased plasma urea (disproportionate to any increase in creatinine)	High-normal/increased plasma sodium
	Normal or decreased plasma sodium	
	Increased haematocrit (not with blood loss)	

Figure 2.4 Features of sodium deficiency and excess

DISTURBANCES OF PLASMA SODIUM CONCENTRATION

It is beyond the scope of this book to discuss this topic in any detail. It cannot be overemphasised that sodium concentration is determined by the amounts of sodium *and* water in the extracellular fluid. Patients with hyponatraemia may have normal, decreased or even increased extracellular fluid contents, and so may appear clinically euvolaemic, hypovolaemic or fluid overloaded (oedematous), respectively. Hypernatraemia can be a consequence of sodium excess or water deficiency. It is thus essential to determine the cause of both hypo- and hyper-natraemia in order to manage these conditions.

ASSESSMENT OF STATUS

The limitations of measuring plasma sodium concentration have been discussed. They must be considered in relation to clinical observations. Measurement of urinary sodium excretion can also be helpful. Because of the considerable ability of the kidneys to conserve sodium, in a hyponatraemic patient a low urinary sodium concentration (<20 mmol/L) suggests sodium depletion. Total body sodium content can be measured using an isotope dilution technique.

Sulphur

Sulphur is present in the amino acids cysteine and methionine. Disulphide linkages play an important part in the secondary structure of proteins and peptide hormones, e.g. insulin. It is also present in collagen and many glycosaminoglycans, e.g. heparan sulphate. Sulphur has an important role in detoxification reactions: sulphation is one of the mechanisms by which fat soluble molecules can be rendered water soluble in the liver, and the antioxidant action of glutathione is a function of its sulphydryl group. The oxidation of sulphur-containing amino acids leads to the formation of sulphuric acid. Sulphate is excreted in urine, as are the buffered hydrogen ions.

Proteins are the major source of dietary sulphur, although inorganic sulphates are also present in the diet.

There is no specific homeostatic mechanism for sulphur or sulphate, nor have any specific syndromes of deficiency or excess of sulphur been described. However, various inherited metabolic diseases involving sulphur-containing compounds, particularly amino acids, have been described (e.g. cystathioninuria); details of these are beyond the scope of this book.

The plasma concentrations of sulphate and sulphur-containing amino acids are amenable to measurement, but there is no indication to do so in routine nutritional practice.

Inorganic micronutrients

Copper

Copper is essential for the activity of several enzymes, including:

- caeruloplasmin – a ferroxidase necessary for the conversion of iron II to iron III in the plasma

- cytochrome c oxidase – terminal step in the electron transport chain

- lysyl oxidase – essential for crosslinking between the polypeptide chains in collagen and elastase

- tyrosinase – involved in the synthesis of melanin

- dopamine hydroxylase – conversion of dopamine to noradrenaline (nor-epinephrine)

- superoxide dismutase – responsible for the destruction of free radicals.

Dietary copper is absorbed in the proximal small gut and transported to the liver, mainly bound to albumin. Here, it is incorporated into caeruloplasmin, which is secreted into the plasma. One molecule of caeruloplasmin contains six copper ions and the protein constitutes about 90% of total plasma copper. An intake of 1.2 mg copper (19 μmol) daily is sufficient to maintain health; cereals, nuts and legumes are good dietary sources. Vitamin C reduces copper absorption by converting it from Cu^{2+} to the less soluble Cu^+ form. It seems paradoxical that vitamin C enhances the absorption of dietary iron, yet reduced availability of copper could impair the utilisation of iron through a reduction in ferroxidase activity.

Deficiency of copper is rare but it has been described in patients with severe malabsorption, malnourished infants and individuals on long-term parenteral nutrition. A high intake of zinc can cause copper deficiency by inducing the synthesis of intestinal metallothionein, which chelates copper and prevents its absorption. The features of copper deficiency include a microcytic anaemia that is unresponsive to iron therapy, neutropenia and osteoporosis. The anaemia may in part be due to unopposed free radical-induced damage to red cell plasma membranes as well as to functional iron deficiency.

Copper can be measured in the plasma (normal range ~11-24 μmol/L) but the results may be confounded by an acute phase response, which increases caeruloplasmin synthesis; measurement of red cell superoxide dismutase provides a better indicator of tissue copper stores. Copper is secreted in bile and can accumulate in the liver in cholestasis. Copper ions are toxic: the ingestion of as little as 20 mg may be sufficient to cause symptoms, which include nausea, vomiting and dizziness.

There are two inherited metabolic disorders involving copper. Wilson's disease is an autosomal recessive condition caused by a defect in a copper-transporting ATPase encoded by the *ATP7B* gene on chromosome 13. Numerous mutations have been found, but one (His1069 → Gly) accounts for about 50% of cases in Western Europe. There is reduced incorporation of copper into caeruloplasmin and accumulation of copper in various tissues, including the liver, kidneys, basal ganglia and corneas. Manifestations of the condition include acute liver failure (particularly in children) and cirrhosis, a Fanconi syndrome, haemolytic anaemia, a neurological disorder that can include tremor, involuntary movements, dysarthria and sometimes dementia, and deposition of copper in Descemet's membrane in the corneas (Kayser-Fleischer rings, a specific sign of the disease). Plasma copper and caeruloplasmin concentrations are usually low and urinary copper increased, often up to ten times normal. Urinary copper excretion is further increased by the administration of pencillamine. Hepatic copper content (measured on biopsy material) is increased but this is not a specific finding. Treatment is with long-term penicillamine, which chelates copper and allows it to be excreted in the urine. Children may be intolerant of penicillamine and an alternative is to give zinc supplements, which reduce copper absorption (see above). The earlier treatment is started, the better the prognosis; the neurological damage is not always reversible. Liver transplantation may be an option in fulminant hepatic failure and end stage chronic liver disease. Members of a patient's family should be screened and treated if found to have the condition, even in the absence of symptoms.

Menke's disease is an X-linked condition that presents in males in early infancy with poor growth, mental retardation and characteristic kinky, brittle hair. It is due to a defect in a gene (*ATP7A*) homologous to the Wilson's gene, which prevents the release of copper from enterocytes into the blood.

Fluorine
The total fluorine content of the body is less than 1 g, of which 99% is in bone, although it is detectable in many tissues. Although fluorine is undoubtedly biologically active, and is known to have positive effects on bone density and dental health, it is uncertain that it is truly an essential nutrient in that no specific syndrome of deficiency has been described. However, the fact that a low fluorine intake is associated with increased risk of dental caries (and of osteoporosis in the

elderly), which can be reduced by fluorine supplementation, has led authorities in many countries to supplement water supplies with fluoride. A water content of 1 ppm (part per million) ensures an intake of 1-2 mg/day and provides an important protective effect without significant risk of toxicity. Fluoridated toothpastes are also a useful source. Fluoride has also been used successfully together with calcium and vitamin D to treat osteoporosis. The mechanism of the protective effect is uncertain.

A water content of more than 3 ppm can cause fluorosis – pitting and discolouration of the teeth in children – although the protection against caries is maintained. In some areas of India, a very high intake leads to increased calcification of bone and even calcification of ligaments and tendons.

Iodine
The only known function of iodine in man is as a constitutent of the two thyroid hormones, thyroxine and triiodothyronine. Seawater contains iodine and seafood provides a rich source of dietary iodine, but vegetables are generally a poor source, except in coastal areas where seawater spray supplies iodine to the soil. Dairy products, eggs and meat are also good sources.

Most dietary iodine is reduced to iodide in the gut prior to absorption. About one third is taken up by the thyroid, and most of the rest is excreted in urine. The recommended intake is 150 µg/day. Iodine deficiency causes decreased synthesis of thyroid hormones, leading to increased secretion of thyroid stimulating hormone, which stimulates the growth of the thyroid (resulting in a visible swelling, or goitre). Iodine deficiency is the most common cause of hypothyroidism worldwide, although it is rare in developed countries. In some mountainous areas of the world where dietary iodine deficiency is widespread, goitre is endemic: patients are not always hypothyroid, however, because the increased thyroid tissue may be able to synthesise adequate quantities of thyroid hormones. Addition of iodine to salt and bread has reduced the number of areas where endemic goitre still occurs. Apparent iodine deficiency is not always a result of a poor intake. Some foods contain substances (goitrogens) that interfere with the utilisation of iodine by the thyroid. Thiocyanates are particularly implicated: they can be formed from glucosinolates during the digestion of certain vegetables (i.e. members of the Cruciferae family – the brassicas) and from cyanogenic glycosides present in cassava, a staple source of carbohydrate in some tropical countries.

A high intake of iodine, such as may occur in individuals eating kelp (seaweed) preparations from 'health food' shops to provide supplementary iodine, is harmful. It can cause goitre and acneiform skin lesions.

Iron

The most important function of iron is as a component of haemoglobin and myoglobin; it is also present in cytochromes and peroxidases. In all these proteins, it is present in haem. Non-haem iron is involved in the activity of several other enzymes, including succinate dehydrogenase, aconitase and phosphoenolpyruvate carboxykinase. Total body iron is about 70 mmol, of which two thirds is in haemoglobin; most of the rest is stored in the reticuloendothelial system as ferritin. Only 0.1% of the total body iron is in the plasma, where almost all is bound to transferrin, its transport protein.

Iron is present in animal products mainly as haem iron and in vegetables mainly as inorganic iron; haem iron is the more readily absorbed form. Much inorganic iron may be unavailable as a result of binding in insoluble complexes, e.g. with phytates and oxalate.

The mean daily intake of iron is about 20 mg (0.36 mmol) but only about 10% is absorbed. The Fe^{2+} form of inorganic iron is more readily absorbed than Fe^{3+}; ascorbic acid promotes iron absorption by reducing Fe^{3+} to Fe^{2+}. The regulation of iron absorption is complex, but in essence it acts to increase iron uptake when body stores are decreased and when there is increased erythropoiesis. Iron is strongly conserved in the body: the obligatory loss in males is only about 18 μmol/day but it is much greater in menstruating women.

Iron deficiency can be dietary in origin, but excess loss is also a major cause. Worldwide, infestation with hookworms is the most common cause. Infants (because of the demands imposed by growth) and women during their reproductive years (because of menstruation and pregnancy) are particularly vulnerable to iron deficiency. Iron deficiency causes a microcytic, hypochromic anaemia. As deficiency develops, depletion of stores leads to a compensatory increase in iron absorption from the gut and anaemia only develops as stores become very low. Other features include brittle nails, koilonychias (spooning of the nails), angular stomatitis, atrophy of the papillae of the tongue and glossitis. The anaemia is characteristic but not pathognomic: other causes of a hypochromic, microcytic anaemia include thalassasemias, sideroblastic anaemia and, sometimes, the anaemia of chronic disease. In these conditions, however, iron stores are usually normal. In iron deficiency anaemia, plasma iron concentration is low and that of transferrin may be increased. Plasma ferritin concentration, reflecting iron stores, is low (typically <20 μg/L), although it can be misleadingly normal during an acute phase response. Plasma soluble transferrin receptor concentrations are increased in iron deficiency, but the rise only occurs after deficiency has developed, whereas ferritin measurement can detect depletion before anaemia has developed. A lack of stainable iron in the bone marrow is diagnostic of iron deficiency, but bone marrow examination is rarely necessary. Iron deficiency usually responds to oral iron (e.g. ferrous gluconate 300 mg twice daily) but it is important to establish whether there is a treatable cause and manage this appropriately. Oral iron should be discontinued once iron stores have been restored, typically after six months' treatment.

Free iron is toxic. Iron poisoning is mainly confined to children who obtain access to iron tablets. It can cause necrosis of the intestinal epithelium, bleeding and fluid loss, and may be complicated by renal and hepatic failure. The specific treatment is with chelating therapy using desferrioxamine.

A chronically high iron intake can lead to iron overload. This can occur in patients requiring repeated blood transfusions, e.g. for thalassemia. The iron initially accumulates in the reticuloendothelial system, where it is harmless, but can eventually become deposited in hepatic parenchymal cells, causing fibrosis, and in the heart. Hereditary haemochromatosis is an inherited (autosomal recessive) disorder of iron metabolism. Most frequently due to a mutation in the *HFE* gene, it results in unregulated absorption of dietary iron and its accumulation in the liver, heart and endocrine tissues. It presents in men in the fourth and fifth decades of life, but much later, if at all, in women. Heterozygotes do not develop significant iron overload.

Haemochromatosis is treated by repeated venesection, but while this usually prevents progression of liver disease, it does not reverse the damage to endocrine organs.

Selenium
In man, selenium is present in at least three enzymes as selenocysteine. These are:

- glutathione peroxidase, an antioxidant enzyme that destroys peroxides, including hydrogen peroxide, using reduced glutathione

- type I iodothyronine 5-deiodinase, which converts thyroxine to triiodothyronine

- thioredoxin reductase, an enzyme involved in nucleotide metabolism.

Other selenoproteins include selenoprotein P, present in the plasma, and selenoprotein W, present in muscle. The function of these proteins is unknown.

Selenium is present in fish, liver and kidneys; the content in vegetables is variable, depending on soil selenium content. The recommended intake for adult men is 75 µg/day.

Selenium deficiency is rare but has been described in patients receiving parenteral nutrition and is the cause of Keshan disease, a cardiomyopathy that occurs in areas of China where the soil content of selenium is low. A skeletal myopathy may also occur.

Epidemiological studies have demonstrated associations between low plasma selenium concentrations and risk of atherosclerotic disease and some cancers, possibly related to a decreased antioxidant activity. Dietary supplementation has been shown to reduce the incidence of some cancers. However, selenium is toxic, and the difference between intakes associated with deficiency and toxicity is unusually small; the daily intake should not exceed 200 µg. The plasma concentration reflects recent intake; measurement of glutathione peroxidase in red blood cells appears to be a better guide to overall selenium status.

Zinc

Zinc is required for many enzymes either structurally or as a cofactor: these include carbonic anhydrase (carbonate dehydratase), alkaline phosphatase (the plasma activity of this enzyme decreases in zinc deficiency), carboxypeptidase, thymidine kinase and enzymes involved in nucleic acid synthesis.

Oysters, eggs, poultry and meat are good dietary sources. Cereals contain significant amounts of zinc, but its bioavailability is limited by the presence of phytates, which bind to it and reduce its absorption. Zinc is absorbed in the proximal small intestine but its release into the bloodstream (where it is bound to albumin) is controlled by metallothionein, a protein whose synthesis is increased when zinc intake is high and falls when it is low. This provides an efficient means for controlling the supply of zinc to the tissues of the body. However, metallothionein also binds copper with a higher affinity, with the result that a high zinc intake can lead to impaired uptake of copper (see p. 45). The recommended intake in adult males is 145 µmol/day (9.4 mg/day). Dietary deficiency is uncommon but is well described, particularly in patients receiving artificial nutrition with inadequate provision. Features include poor wound healing, defective immune function, anorexia, ageusia (decreased sense of taste) and dermatitis. Severe zinc deficiency is seen in acrodermatitis enteropathica, an inherited disorder caused by malabsorption of zinc. This is a severe, primarily acral, dermatitis. The condition is fatal if untreated but responds rapidly to zinc replacement.

Zinc is generally less toxic than other metallic micronutrients, but toxicity has been reported in relation to the storage of water in galvanised containers. Features include gastrointestinal disturbances and, as mentioned above, a risk of copper deficiency.

Zinc can readily be measured in plasma but the fact that it is largely bound to albumin in the plasma should be borne in mind when interpreting the results. The normal concentration is 10-20 µmol/L.

Other inorganic micronutrients

Deficiency syndromes of three other elements, chromium, manganese and molybdenum, have been reported, but only in subjects receiving artificial forms of nutrition (Figure 2.5). The human body also contains several other elements, including silicon, boron, nickel, vanadium, arsenic and tin. Deficiency diseases for some of these have been described in animals, but there is no firm evidence that any is essential for health in man.

Other inorganic micronutrients

Element	Roles	Comments
Chromium	Present in glucose tolerance factor – important for binding of insulin to receptors	Deficiency causes impaired glucose tolerance
	Lipoprotein metabolism	Supplementation reported to reduce plasma cholesterol and triglyceride concentrations
Manganese	Present in pyruvate carboxylase, superoxide dismutase, glycosyl transferase and arginase	Deficiency rarely described: features include weight loss and dermatitis, and falls in plasma cholesterol and triglyceride concentrations
		Toxicity causes cholestasis and movement disorder. It has been described in miners (from inhalation), children receiving parenteral nutrition and in areas of the world where there is a high concentration in water
Molybdenum	Cofactor for aldehyde oxidase, xanthine oxidase and sulphite oxidase	Deficiency rarely described: causes headache, lethargy, coma

Figure 2.5 Other inorganic micronutrients

Organic micronutrients

The vitamins are a disparate group of organic compounds that are essential for normal metabolism and, because they cannot be synthesised to any extent in the body, are essential components of a healthy diet. The name derives from the term 'vital amines' but this is clearly a misnomer since none of them is an amine.

They are conventionally divided into two groups – the water soluble vitamins (B and C) and fat soluble vitamins (A, D, E and K). The astute reader will note that some letters between A and K are missing: there are various reasons for this. For example, letter H was originally assigned to a water soluble substance later identified as biotin and now included within the B group; likewise, vitamin G, riboflavin, is now assigned to the B group; the letter F was given to what are now known to be the essential fatty acids. Letter B is assigned to a group of water soluble vitamins: vitamin B_{12} is cobalamin, but usually referred to as vitamin B_{12}; vitamins B_1 and B_2 are thiamin and riboflavin, respectively, and are usually referred to by name. Folic acid is vitamin B_9, but is invariably referred to by name, as is vitamin B_7 (biotin).

The grouping together of the various B vitamins reflects their function as components of coenzymes or prosthetic groups; vitamin C, although also water soluble, has unrelated metabolic functions. Apart from their essential status (not absolute in the case of vitamin D), the only property that the fat soluble vitamins have in common is their hydrophobicity.

Vitamin A

FUNCTION
Vitamin A is retinol, an unsaturated long chain alcohol attached to a β-ionone ring (Figure 2.6); the latter is essential for its activity. Retinol and related compounds have three major functions:

- 11-*cis*-retinal is present in the opsin proteins of rods (rhodopsin, visual purple) and cones (iodopsins) of the retina. Light causes retinal to be converted to its *trans*-isomer and released from its opsin, triggering changes in membrane potentials that are relayed to the brain. Regeneration of rhodopsin involves isomerisation of *cis*-retinal and recombination with opsin (Figure 2.7)

- retinyl phosphate is a cofactor in the synthesis of mannose-containing glycoproteins

- retinol and retinoic acid are involved in the control of the differentiation and proliferation of epithelial and other (notably bone) cells. They are required for normal epithelial cell function, including mucin secretion, and for bone growth.

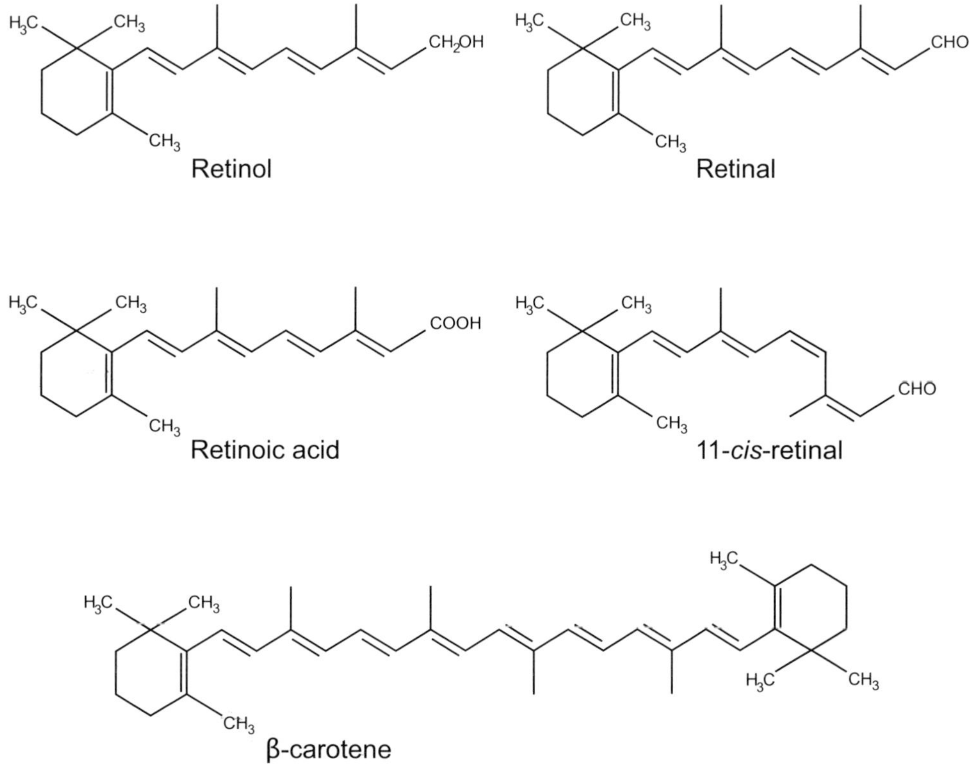

Figure 2.6 The structures of retinol and other retinoids.

SOURCES, TRANSPORT AND METABOLISM

Retinol is present in food mainly in the form of esters, particularly with palmitic acid. Absorption from the gut involves hydrolysis and re-esterification in enterocytes, whence it is transported in chylomicrons and stored in the liver. The richest food source is liver; fish oils, egg yolks and milk are other good sources. Retinol can be made in the body from some carotenoids, of which the most important is β-carotene; these are plant products, which occur particularly in carrots and green vegetables. β-Carotene is converted to retinal in enterocytes by oxidative cleavage; reduction of retinal by alcohol dehydrogenase yields retinol. The recommended daily intake of vitamin A is 700 μg/day.

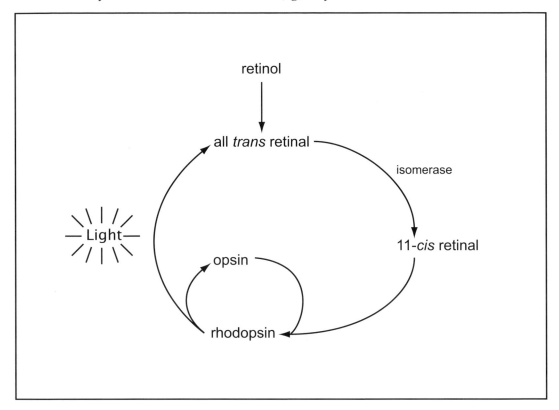

Figure 2.7 The visual cycle, showing the effect of light on rhodopsin, and its regeneration.

Carotene provides approximately a quarter of dietary vitamin A in the UK. Although each molecule of carotene would appear to yield two molecules of retinal, the actual yield is less: 6 μg of carotene is equivalent to 1 μg of retinal, and hence retinol.

Retinol is released from the liver bound to retinol-binding protein and transported to tissues in a protein-protein complex with prealbumin. If the concentrations of these proteins are reduced by malnutrition, failure of delivery of vitamin A to peripheral tissues can cause decreased plasma concentrations even if there are adequate hepatic stores of the vitamin.

THE BIOCHEMISTRY AND PHYSIOLOGY OF INDIVIDUAL NUTRIENTS

DEFICIENCY

The rods of the retina are responsible for perceiving dim light. It is for this reason that deficiency of vitamin A causes defective night vision (nyctalopia). More importantly, deficiency causes xerophthalmia, keratinisation of the conjunctivae with drying of the eye leading to corneal degeneration (keratomalacia) and blindness. Night blindness is reversible: corneal degeneration is not. The latter may be complicated by infection, which may contribute to loss of sight. Vitamin A deficiency is a major cause of blindness in the world, particularly among children. Other effects of deficiency include poor growth of bones and teeth and increased susceptibility to infections, particularly respiratory. Vitamin A deficiency is treated with 30 mg retinyl palmitate for two days. If necessary, 30 mg may be given parenterally.

EXCESS

Vitamin A is toxic in excess. Both high single doses and a chronically high intake can be harmful: features of the latter include coarsening and loss of hair, dermatoses and bone fragility. It is also teratogenic (though β-carotene is not).

ASSESSMENT OF STATUS

The normal plasma concentration of retinol is 1-2.5 μmol/L. However, facilities for its measurement are rarely available in areas of the world where deficiency is common, so the diagnosis is usually made clinically and confirmed retrospectively by the response to treatment.

The B vitamins

The major properties of the B vitamins are summarised in Figure 2.8. In developed countries, isolated deficiency of B vitamins (with the exception of folate and vitamin B_{12}, and, less frequently, thiamin and niacin) is uncommon. The B vitamins are in general non-toxic in excess, presumably because they are water soluble and readily excreted in the urine: an exception is pyridoxine, a high intake of which can cause (reversible) peripheral neuropathy. It can also interfere with the action of levodopa in patients treated for Parkinson's disease. With the exception of vitamin B_{12}, the body stores only limited quantities of most water soluble vitamins.

SOURCES

The B vitamins are present in a wide variety of foods of both animal and vegetable origin, with the exception of vitamin B_{12}, which is confined to the animal kingdom (including yeasts). However, there is variation: for example, green leafy vegetables are a particularly good source of folic acid; in grain, thiamin is largely present in the germ and outer coat of the seed, and considerable loss takes place during milling.

Water soluble vitamins

Vitamin B₁ (thiamin)

Active form

Thiamin pyrophosphate

Major functions

Coenzyme for;
- decarboxylations (e.g. pyruvate to acetyl CoA, α-oxoglutarate to succinyl CoA)
- transketolation in phosphogluconate pathway (required for synthesis of pentoses and production of reduced NADPH – itself required, e.g. for cholesterol synthesis)
- metabolism of branched chain amino acids

Recommended daily intake*

0.5 mg/1000 kcals. In deficiency, 50 mg parenterally daily for three days, then 25 mg orally

Effects of deficiency

Beri-beri: the earliest feature is peripheral neuropathy (dry beri-beri); later, in chronic deficiency, cardiac failure leads to oedema (wet beri-beri); severe acute deficiency causes the Wernicke-Korsakoff syndrome, with early confusion leading to loss of recent memory, confabulation, abnormal eye movements and peripheral neuropathy. This is a medical emergency.

Vitamin B₂ (riboflavin)

Active form

Riboflavin mononucleotide (FMN); dinucleotide (FAD)

Major functions

Prosthetic groups for oxidation-reduction reactions in numerous metabolic pathways, e.g.
- cytochrome c reductase
- succinyl CoA dehydrogenase
- glutathione reductase

Recommended daily intake*

1.3 mg daily

Effects of deficiency

No specific deficiency syndrome has been described, and when riboflavin deficiency does occur it is often associated with deficiencies of other nutrients. Features seen in deficiency include angular stomatitis, a red inflamed tongue, seborrhoeic dermatitis and corneal vascularisation and lens opacity.

Notes

Riboflavin is present in vegetables and animal products. Assessment of status is possible by measuring plasma concentration (normal 120-160 nmol/L).Tissue stores are better assessed by measuring the activity of red cell glutathione reductase.

Figure 2.8 Water soluble vitamins
* in adult males: greater amounts are required in children, during pregnancy and illness

Water soluble vitamins (cont.)

Niacin (nicotinic acid and nicotinamide)

Active form Nicotinamide adenine dinucleotide (NAD) and its phosphate (NADP)

Major functions NAD and NADP act as hydrogen acceptors in numerous oxidative reactions, and hydrogen donors in reductive reactions.

Recommended daily intake* 6.6 mg/1000 kcal energy/day
In deficiency: 300 mg daily orally

Effects of deficiency Pellagra: in severe cases, this comprises dermatitis, diarrhoea and dementia, but in mild cases only glossitis, with a burning pain in the oral cavity, may be present. Deficiency may be caused by treatment with isoniazid, which can cause deficiency of vitamin B_6, needed for synthesis of nicotinamide from tryptophan.

Notes Diagnosis is based on the clinical features, although because deficiencies of other B vitamins can cause similar changes, and other deficiencies may be present, treatment is usually with a multivitamin mixture.

Vitamin B_6 (occurs as pyridoxine, pyridoxal and pyridoxamine)

Active form Pyridoxal 5-phosphate

Major functions Coenzyme for more than 60 enzymes, many of which are involved in the metabolism of amino acids (including the formation of 5-hydroxy-tryptamine from tryptophan) and also the synthesis of δ-amino-laevulinic acid, the rate limiting step of porphyrin synthesis.

Recommended daily intake* 15 μg/g dietary protein

Effects of deficiency The vitamin is widespread in foodstuffs and dietary deficiency is very rare. Deficiency can cause glossitis and polyneuropathy. A sideroblastic anaemia has been described in chronic alcoholics that is associated with low plasma concentration of the vitamin and responds to supplementation. Various drugs (e.g. isoniazid and penicillamine) are antagonists of the vitamin, which should be given prophylactically to avoid deficiency when these drugs are used.

Notes Several genetic B_6-dependent syndromes have been described including a sideroblastic anaemia due to defective δ-aminolaevulinic acid synthetase, and some forms of homocystinuria. Pharmacological doses of vitamin B_6 are sometimes used in the treatment of pre-menstrual tension and other conditions, but a chronically high intake can increase normal requirements (thus risking deficiency on cessation) and cause a polyneuropathy.

Water soluble vitamins (cont.)

Biotin

Active form	Biotin
Major functions	Biotin acts as a prosthetic group for four carboxylase enzymes, including pyruvate and acetyl CoA carboxylases.
Recommended daily intake*	50-100 µg/day
Effects of deficiency	Deficiency (manifest as a dermatitis) is very rare. It is a potential problem if raw eggs are consumed in quantity: they contain avidin, a glycoprotein that binds biotin with high affinity.

Pantothenic acid

Active form	Coenzyme A
Major functions	Coenzyme A is essential for the metabolism of carbohydrates, fats and proteins. The combination of acetyl CoA with oxaloacetate to yield citrate is the first reaction in the tricarboxylic acid (citric acid, Krebs) cycle.
Recommended daily intake	4-7 mg/day
Effects of deficiency	Despite its key function in intermediary metabolism, no specific naturally occurring deficiency syndrome is described. Experimentally induced deficiency causes numerous symptoms and signs, including painful peripheral neuropathy.

Vitamin B$_{12}$

Active form	Methyl- and deoxyadenosyl-cobalamins
Major functions	• Coenzyme for conversion of folic acid to active form • Coenzyme for metabolism of methylmalonate to succinate
Recommended daily intake*	2.0 µg/day (4.0 in pregnancy and lactation). For treatment of deficiency: 1000 µg i.m as hydroxycobalamin every three months once body stores replete
Effects of deficiency	• Macrocytic, megaloblastic anaemia • Neurological disorder
Notes	Normal plasma concentration 250-900 ng/L

Water soluble vitamins (cont.)

Folic acid

Active form	Tetrahydrofolic acid
Major functions	Single carbon transfers: • in purine and pyrimidine synthesis • in the interconversions of: histidine-glutamate; serine-glycine; homocysteine-methionine • conversion of deoxyuridylate to deoxythymidylate (hence DNA synthesis)
Recommended daily intake*	200 µg/day (supplements recommended during pregnancy and lactation). In deficiency: 5 mg daily for three months
Effects of deficiency	Macrocytosis, megaloblastic anaemia
Notes	Normal plasma concentration 3-13 µg/L: red cell 180-750 µg/L; red cell concentration is a better indicator of tissue folate status; in vitamin B_{12} deficiency plasma folate concentration tends to rise while red cell concentration falls. Folic acid supplements may lower plasma concentrations of homocysteine (a risk factor for cardiovascular disease) but there is no consistent evidence that doing so is beneficial.

ASSESSMENT OF STATUS

A variety of techniques have been employed in the past to assess the body's content of B vitamins, including measurements of the vitamins themselves, the measurement of metabolites in the urine and functional assays, in which the activity of an enzyme for which the vitamin is a cofactor is measured (e.g. red cell transketolase for thiamin). Specific assays now exist for the measurement of all the B vitamins in plasma and, in the case of folate, in red blood cells. However, with the exception of folate and vitamin B_{12}, it is rarely necessary formally to assess B vitamin status. These two apart, if deficiency is suspected, a multivitamin preparation can be given and the clinical response monitored. If thiamin deficiency is suspected or anticipated (see p.60) thiamin must be given as a matter of urgency to prevent the development of encephalopathy.

Individual B vitamins

THIAMIN

Thiamin has a central role in intermediary metabolism, particularly of carbohydrates. Thiamin deficiency is a potential problem in two particular groups of patients – chronic alcoholics, whose food intake may be very poor, and those with malnutrition secondary to any cause of inadequate food intake. In the latter, clinical evidence of thiamin deficiency may become apparent on refeeding, owing to the high thiamin requirement imposed by increased energy intake in the form of glucose. Deficiency should be anticipated in both circumstances and parenteral thiamin (100 mg) administered to prevent the development of the Wernicke-Korsakoff syndrome, some components of which may rapidly become irreversible.

NIACIN

The clinical features of niacin deficiency (see Figure 2.8) may occasionally be a part of carcinoid syndrome. Some of the body's nicotinic acid is derived from the endogenous metabolism of tryptophan, and in carcinoid, increased production of 5-hydroxytryptamine from this precursor may reduce the formation of niacin to the extent that dietary intake alone is insufficient to maintain adequate body stores.

FOLATE

Structure and function
Folic acid comprises pteroylglutamic acid: pteridine linked through *p*-aminobenzoic acid to glutamic acid (Figure 2.9). In food, it is present mainly as polyglutamates, but the extra glutamate residues are removed at the surface of enterocytes before absorption. Most then undergoes methylation and reduction to tetrahydromethylfolate, the major form of the vitamin in the circulation, although in tissues it is stored as polyglutamates.

Folic acid itself has no biological activity: the active forms are di- and tetrahydrofolates, which act as donors and acceptors of 1-carbon groups (e.g. methyl, methenyl, formyl and methylene) in reactions including the interconversion of certain amino acids (see Figure 2.8) and the formation of thymidylate from deoxyuridylate, an essential reaction in purine (and thus DNA) synthesis.

Deficiency
Deficiency of folate can be due to dietary insufficiency (rare in developed countries), malabsorption, excess utilisation (e.g. during lactation) or loss (e.g. during dialysis). The characteristic consequence is a macrocytic, megaloblastic anaemia,

which responds rapidly to folate supplementation. The relationship with vitamin B_{12} is considered in the next section. In addition, some drugs, e.g. methotrexate, pyrimethamine and trimethoprim, antagonise the effects of folate (Figure 2.9: see next section). Phenytoin may decrease the intestinal absorption of folate, as may alcohol, which also increases renal folate excretion: a raised mean cell volume is a common finding in people abusing alcohol.

Dietary supplementation (400 µg daily) with folate from the time of conception to the twelfth week of pregnancy has been proven to reduce the incidence of neural tube defects. A partial deficiency of the enzyme methyltetrahydrofolate reductase has been reported in some parents of infants born with such defects. Women who have had a child with a neural tube defect should take 5 mg folic acid daily before and during any subsequent pregnancy. Folate prophylaxis is also recommended in chronic haematological disorders, e.g. β-thalassaemias and haemolytic conditions, in which there is increased red cell turnover.

Folate deficiency is treated with folic acid 5 mg daily: a four month course is sufficient to replenish body stores provided that the underlying cause can be treated successfully.

Folate antagonists
Folate antagonists are used therapeutically in chemotherapy and as antimicrobials. They act by competing for the enzyme dihydrofolate reductase, preventing the formation of tetrahydrofolate. Methotrexate is a powerful inhibitor of this enzyme and inhibits purine synthesis in cancer cells. A high dose is infused intravenously, the rationale being that a high concentration for a short time will kill cancer cells but spare other tissues. However, it may affect the bone marrow, and the finding of too high a plasma concentration of methotrexate following infusion is an indication to give folinic acid as a source of folate to protect the marrow. A concentration of >5.0 µmol/L at 24 h or >0.5 µmol/L at 48 h after the infusion is an indication to do this. Antimicrobial folate antagonists (e.g. trimethoprim) are not prone to this complication, as they act selectively against the microbial enzymes.

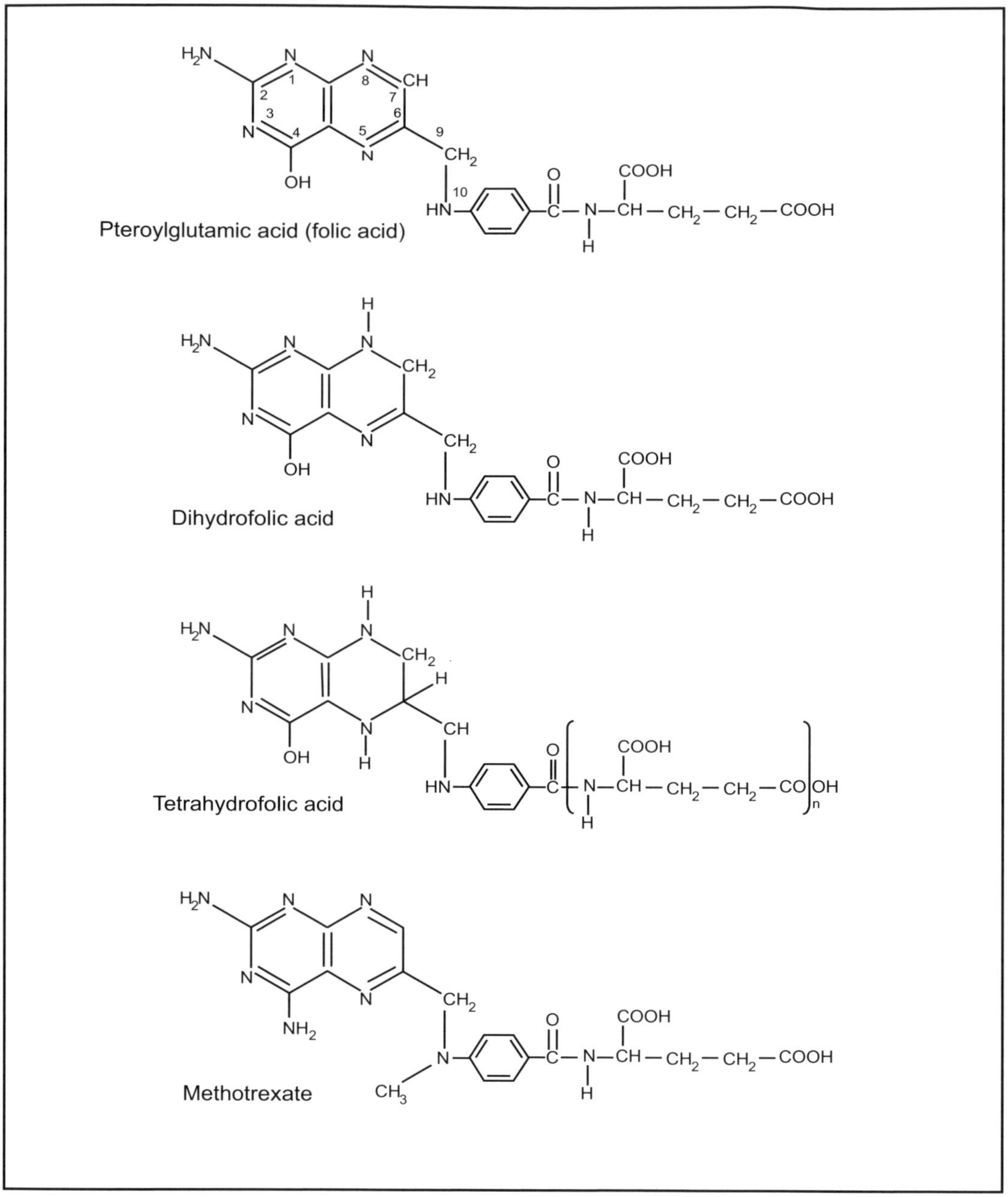

Figure 2.9 The structures of folic acids, dihydrofolic acid and tetrahydrofolic acid (shown as polyglutamate). Folate takes part in single-carbon transfers, involving substitutions at the 5 and 10 positions (see Figure 2.11). Also shown is methotrexate, an antimetabolite that has considerable structural homology with dihydrofolate and is a competitive inhibitor for dihydrofolate reductase.

VITAMIN B$_{12}$

Structure and function
Vitamin B$_{12}$ is a cobalamin, a family of compounds consisting of a planar, cobalt containing (corrin) ring and a ribonucleotide set at a right angle and bound covalently to the ring with a coordinate linkage to the cobalt ion (Figure 2.10). It is of interest that this is the only known example of a carbon-metal bond in a biologically active molecule. There are several different forms of the vitamin, which differ in the ligand to cobalt opposite the nucleotide: the major form in the plasma is methylcobalamin, others being hydroxocobalamin and deoxyadenosylcobalamin.

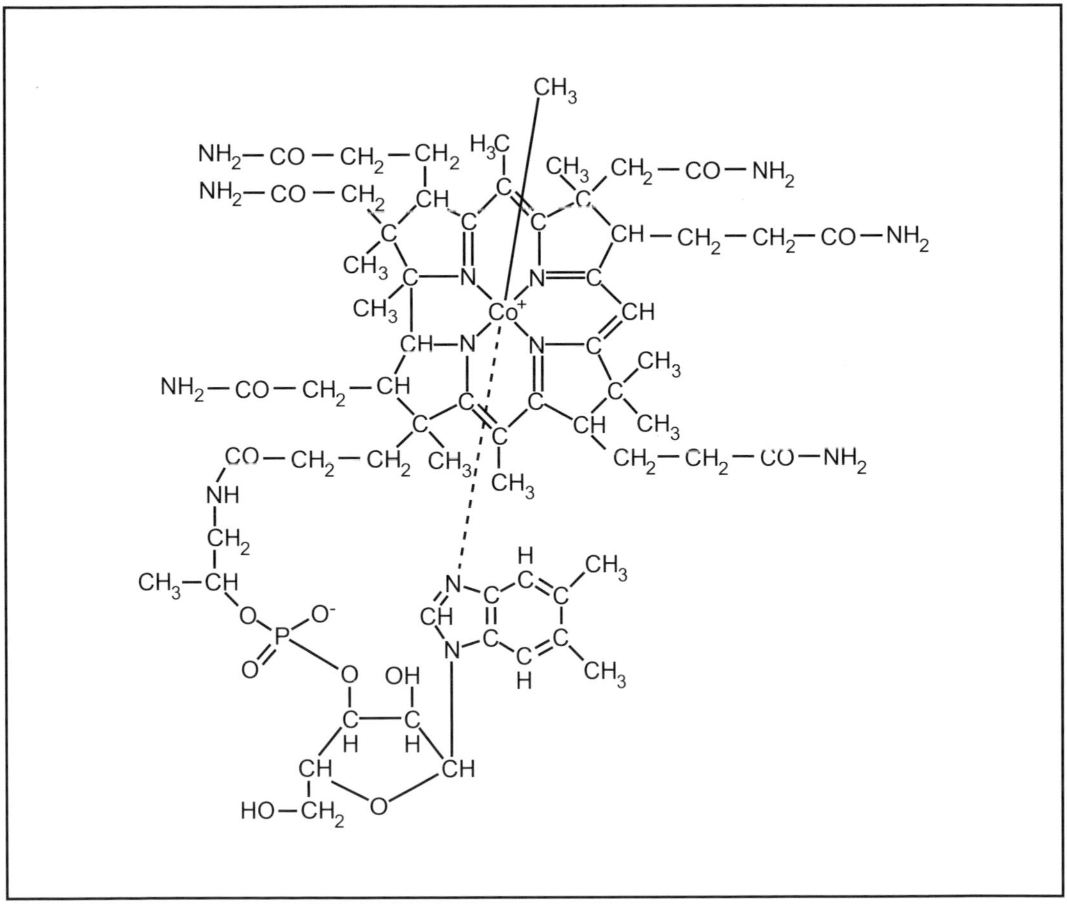

Figure 2.10 Vitamin B$_{12}$. Methylcobalamin, the major circulating form is shown. The ribonucleotide is set at a right angle to the planar corrin ring. The active substituent (methyl or deoxyadenosine) is situated on the other side of the ring.

Vitamin B_{12} is an essential coenzyme for the conversion of homocysteine and methyltetrahydrofolate to methionine and tetrahydrofolate, and is essential to the synthesis of DNA (Figure 2.11). In addition, deoxyadenosylcobalamin is a co-enzyme for methylmalonate CoA mutase, the enzyme responsible for the conversion of methylmalonyl CoA to succinyl CoA. Supplementation is of benefit in some patients with methylmalonic acidaemia, in which there is an inherited deficiency of the enzyme.

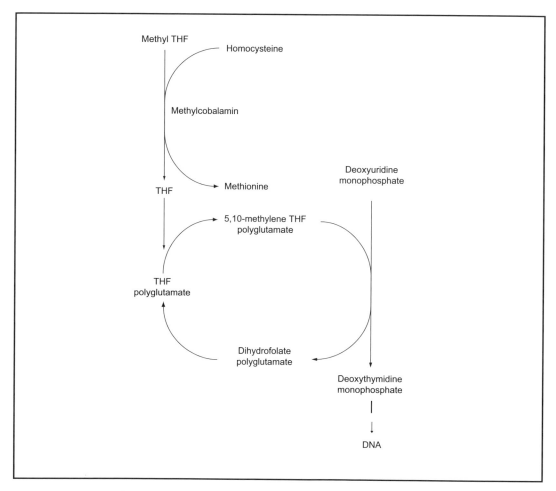

Figure 2.11 The relationship between folate and vitamin B_{12}. 5,10-methyleneTHF polyglutamate is essential for the conversion of deoxyuridine monophosphate to deoxythymidine monophosphate, a step in DNA synthesis. The formation of 5,10-methyleneTHF polyglutamate from methylTHF polyglutamate (the major circulating form of folate) requires the methylcobalamin-dependent conversion of homocysteine to methionine.
THF = tetrahydrofolate

Sources

Vitamin B_{12} is confined to the animal kingdom: meat (especially liver), eggs and milk are good sources. Normal adult stores of the vitamin, in the liver, are 2-3 mg but daily losses are small and features of deficiency may take more than a year to become apparent. Vegans are at risk of vitamin B_{12} deficiency but may obtain sufficient from soil bacteria contaminating their food. The major causes of deficiency are pernicious anaemia (see p.100) and malabsorption.

Absorption and transport

The absorption of vitamin B_{12} is discussed in Chapter 3. In the plasma, it is transported to tissues by a carrier protein, transcobalamin II. Two other transcobalamins (I and III) are also present in the plasma; these may have a role in storage but do not appear to have a role in transport to dividing cells. The majority of vitamin B_{12} in the plasma is bound to transcobalamin I.

Deficiency

Vitamin B_{12} deficiency causes two major clinical conditions: a macrocytic, mega loblastic anaemia, and a neurological disorder, typically beginning with a peripheral neuropathy and progressing to affect the spinal cord, particularly the dorsal and later the lateral columns (subacute combined degeneration). Left untreated, these may be irreversible. Dementia and psychiatric symptoms may also ensue with long-term deficiency.

Vitamin B_{12} deficiency is usually diagnosed on the basis of the clinical evidence and low plasma concentrations (<200 ng/L), although assay results can sometimes be misleading (Figure 2.12). Determining whether a megaloblastic anaemia is caused by folate or vitamin B_{12} deficiency is essential: giving large doses of folate alone in marginal B_{12} deficiency can exacerbate the neuropathy. Occasionally, in an acutely ill patient, treatment may need to be begun before the results of plasma concentrations are available: both vitamins should then be given. Vitamin B_{12} is given as hydroxocobalamin 1000 µg i.m. twice weekly for three weeks, and every three months thereafter. In pernicious anaemia, and in patients with acquired deficiency of intrinsic factor following gastrectomy, treatment must be lifelong.

Vitamin B_{12}, folic acid and homocysteine

A high concentration of the amino acid homocysteine in the blood is an independent risk factor for cardiovascular disease. It is estimated that an increase in concentration of 5 µmol/L (normal 5-12 µmol/L) doubles an individual's risk. Homocystinuria, an inherited metabolic disorder in which plasma concentrations of homocysteine are very high, is a cause of premature cardiovascular disease and thrombosis. Folic acid and vitamins B_6 and B_{12} are all involved in homocysteine metabolism (the roles of folate and B_{12} have been discussed above; cystathionine β-synthase, which catalyses the conversion of homocysteine to cystathionine, is a B_6-dependent enzyme).

It has been demonstrated that treatment with these three vitamins can reduce plasma homocysteine concentrations and in one study this was associated with a decrease in the rate of restenosis after coronary angioplasty. However, results from another trial demonstrated an increase in the rate of restenosis in patients treated by stenting.

Typical laboratory findings in vitamin B_{12} deficiency

Investigation	Results
Full blood count	Anaemia; raised mean cell volume
Peripheral blood film	Macrocytosis; hypersegmented neutrophils
Bone marrow	Megaloblastic erythropoiesis
Serum bilirubin	Elevated (unconjugated)
Serum vitamin B_{12}	Low
Serum folate	Normal or high
Red cell folate	Normal or low

Figure 2.12 Typical laboratory findings in vitamin B_{12} deficiency

Vitamin C

Vitamin C is L-ascorbic acid (Figure 2.13). Its deficiency disease, scurvy, is described in Egyptian writing surviving from 1500 BC. It has an enduring place in history: many military campaigns and exploratory expeditions were affected by the development of scurvy in the participants. In the 18th century, James Lind, a British naval medical officer, conducted possibly the first recorded clinical trial and demonstrated that the provision of oranges to sailors prevented the development of the disease. James Cook demonstrated that the provision of fresh fruit and vegetables to sailors on long voyages prevented the development of scurvy, and the British navy introduced lemon juice rations throughout its fleet, which contributed materially to the better health of British crews in comparison to that of their French and Spanish opponents, and to the ultimate supremacy of the Royal Navy in the Napoleonic Wars.

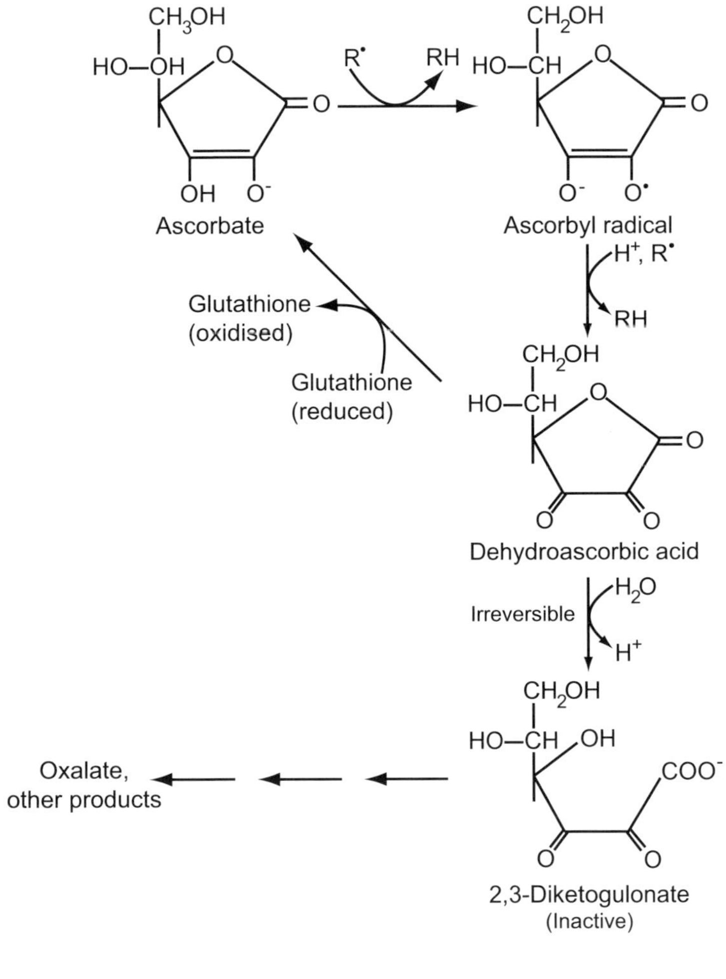

Figure 2.13 Vitamin C (L-ascorbic acid) and its role in scavenging free radicals. Dehydroascorbic acid can be metabolised to oxalate or reduced to ascorbate by glutathione.

R• indicates a free radical

FUNCTION

Unlike the B vitamins, ascorbic acid does not function as a specific coenzyme. A powerful reducing agent, its major function appears to be in controlling the redox potential within cells, acting as an antioxidant and scavenger of free radicals (see Figure 2.13). It is involved in several hydroxylation reactions and is essential to the formation of collagen. The cross-linking of the three polypeptide chains of which mature collagen is composed depends on the post-translational hydroxylation of lysine and proline by lysyl and prolyl hydroxylases. These are iron II- (Fe^{2+}) dependent enzymes, and ascorbate is required to maintain iron in the reduced state. It also has a role in the synthesis of carnitine (required for the transport of fatty acyl CoAs into mitochondria for oxidation), serotonin, dopamine and bile salts.

In the gut, ascorbate promotes the absorption of inorganic iron by maintaining it in the reduced (iron II) state; it may protect against cancer by inhibiting the formation of nitrosamines from nitrite.

SOURCES

Ascorbic acid is widely distributed in the vegetable kingdom, particularly in citrus fruits, tomatoes and leafy vegetables. Root vegetables are relatively low in vitamin C but potatoes are an important source for many people because they are consumed in large quantities. It is of interest that most animals can synthesise ascorbic acid from glucose. Man shares the inability to do so with primates, cavies (guinea-pigs), fruit-eating bats and bul-bul birds: all lack the enzyme L-gulonolactone oxidase required for this process. The recommended intake for adults is 40 mg/day.

DEFICIENCY

Scurvy is characterised by perifollicular haemorrhages, swollen gums with loosening of the teeth, easy bruising, spontaneous haemorrhage, failure of wound healing and anaemia (usually hypochromic unless there is associated haematinic deficiency). These may be preceded by non-specific weakness and myalgia. In infants, subperiosteal haemorrhages, particularly affecting the ends of the long bones, are typical and the limbs are painful as a result. Symptoms take 2-3 months to develop following change to an ascorbate-free diet. Deficiency is simply treated by giving ascorbate 250 mg/day initially until the clinical features have regressed, then ensuring an intake of 40 mg/day. Although widely promulgated as a means of preventing various ailments, particularly the common cold, but also cancer and atherosclerosis, there is no evidence that a high intake (e.g. 1000 mg/day) is effective for these purposes. It may be noted that intestinal absorption is saturable at 1-2 g/day and that excess ascorbate is readily excreted in the urine.

ASSESSMENT OF STATUS

Although clinical scurvy is rare in the UK (and the presentation is usually characteristic), sub-clinical deficiency is probably relatively common, and confirmation may be required. Normal plasma concentrations are about 25-50 µmol/L; in clinically obvious deficiency, concentrations of <10 µmol/L are typical.

Tissue ascorbate concentration is better reflected by measurement in the buffy coat layer (white cells and platelets) on centrifugation of whole blood: this is normally 1.1-3.8 pmol/10^6 cells. Measurement of urine ascorbate after an oral dose of 500 mg (retained in deficiency, >50 % excreted in 24 h in healthy individuals) is an alternative.

Vitamin D

The term vitamin D comprises two secosterols, ergocalciferol (vitamin D_2) and cholecalciferol (vitamin D_3). Ergocalciferol is semi-synthetic, and the form present in foods fortified with vitamin D. Cholecalciferol is produced by the action of ultraviolet radiation from sunlight on 7-dehydrocholesterol in the skin (Figure 2.14). The metabolism and action of the two forms of the vitamin are effectively the same. Since cholecalciferol is the major circulating form, this term is used to denote both in the following account.

SOURCES AND METABOLISM

Cholecalciferol is present in dairy products and egg yolk but, in general, food (especially vegetables) is a poor source and endogenous synthesis provides the major source of the vitamin for most people. Cholecalciferol has no biological activity. It undergoes rapid metabolism in the liver to 25-hydroxycholecalciferol, which is transported in the blood bound to an α_2-globulin and is the major circulating form of the vitamin. 25-hydroxycholecalciferol is further metabolised in the kidney, either to 1,25-dihydroxycholecalciferol (also known as calcitriol) or 24,25-dihydroxycholecalciferol. Calcitriol is a calcium-regulating hormone; 24,25-dihydroxycholecalciferol is biologically inactive. The formation of calcitriol is stimulated by parathyroid hormone and hypophosphataemia and inhibited by calcitriol itself.

FUNCTION

The principal actions of calcitriol are to stimulate the absorption of calcium and phosphate from the gut; it acts on bone synergistically with parathyroid hormone to stimulate osteoclastic bone breakdown, which in turn stimulates new bone formation, and has a minor action in the kidneys to stimulate the reabsorption of filtered calcium. Its overall action is primarily to maintain the plasma calcium concentration at a level that is optimal for bone mineralisation. However, it also has actions apparently unrelated to its effects on calcium metabolism, being involved in the differentiation of cells of the immune system.

DEFICIENCY

Deficiency of vitamin D in children causes rickets, a disorder of impaired bone mineralisation. Bones become soft and deformable. Permanent deformity may occur if the condition is not recognised and treated promptly. The corresponding condition in adults is osteomalacia, characterised by increased osteoid width. Deformity is uncommon but pathological fractures may occur. In both infants and adults there may be bone pain and tenderness, and a sometimes severe proximal myopathy. Vitamin D deficiency can be caused by dietary deficiency, especially in individuals who have low exposure to sunlight (e.g. the elderly), and by malabsorption. Some anticonvulsants induce hepatic enzymes that degrade vitamin D and its metabolites and can cause osteomalacia. Calcitriol concentrations are decreased in patients with chronic renal failure, primarily as a result of the phosphate retention, and this contributes to the pathogenesis of renal osteodystrophy. The homeostatic response to the fall in calcium concentration that occurs in vitamin D deficiency is an increase in the secretion of parathyroid hormone (secondary hyperparathyroidism).

There are two inherited disorders related to the action of vitamin D: vitamin D-dependent rickets types I and II. The inheritance of both is autosomal dominant. In type I, there is decreased 1-hydroxylation of 25-hydroxycholecalciferol; in type II, the defect is in the calcitriol receptor.

EXCESS

Excessive exposure to sunlight does not cause vitamin D toxicity, as cholecalciferol undergoes light-induced isomerisation to inactive metabolites. Furthermore, the formation of calcitriol is tightly regulated by negative feedback inhibition. However, plasma 25-hydroxycholecalciferol concentrations tend to be higher in the summer, and in patients with sarcoidosis and certain other disorders (in whom the 1-hydroxylation reaction is not subject to metabolic control), hypercalcaemia can occur, and does so more frequently during the summer. 25-hydroxycholecalciferol does have some biological activity and a high oral intake of vitamin D can cause hypercalcaemia; if maintained, this can lead to metastatic calcification.

ASSESSMENT OF STATUS

Vitamin D status is assessed by measuring plasma 25-hydroxycholecalciferol concentration (normal 50-150 nmol/L); assays for calcitriol are also available but though indicating the amount of the active form of the vitamin, they do not reflect body stores.

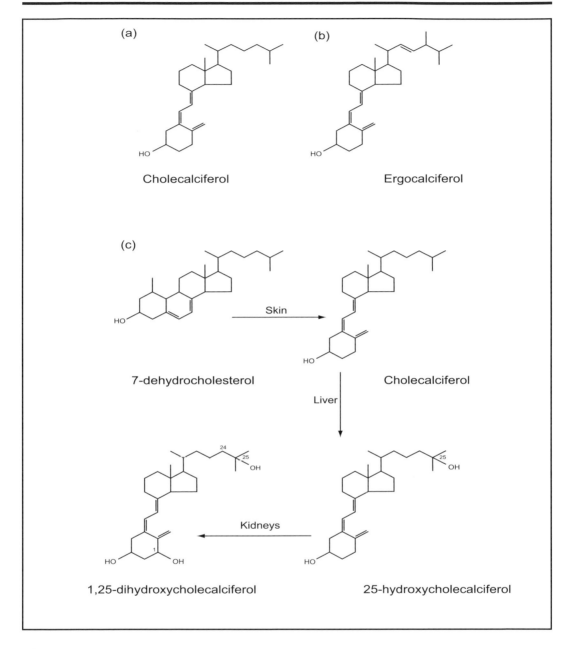

Figure 2.14

a. Cholecalciferol (vitamin D$_3$)

b. Ergocalciferol (vitamin D$_2$)

c. The formation of cholecalciferol from 7-dehydrocholesterol and its subsequent conversion to calcitriol by 25-hydroxylation in the liver and 1-hydroxylation in the kidneys

Vitamin E

The term vitamin E encompasses a group of eight substances, each of which has a 6-chromanol ring structure and a side chain. The four tocopherols (α, β, γ and δ) have saturated side chains; the four tocotrienols have similar side chains except for being unsaturated in the 3', 7' and 11' positions (Figure 2.15). α-Tocopherol is the most abundant and biologically active form; β-tocopherol has a potency about 50% that of α-tocopherol; the tocotrienols make little contribution to overall vitamin E activity.

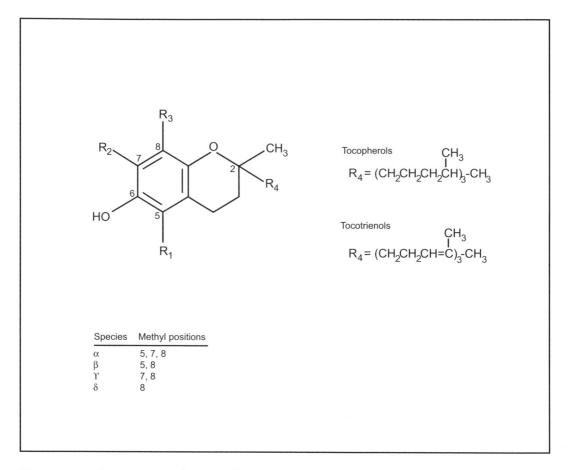

Species	Methyl positions
α	5, 7, 8
β	5, 8
γ	7, 8
δ	8

Figure 2.15 Structures of naturally occurring species of vitamin E

FUNCTION AND SOURCES

Vitamin E is a powerful antioxidant, and this appears to be the basis of its principal biological activity. Being fat soluble, it is particularly important in protecting lipids, including cell membranes, from oxidative damage.

The requirement for vitamin E has not been precisely defined; it is increased by a high intake of polyunsaturated fatty acids, which are more easily oxidised. With a normal diet, an intake of 10 mg per day is probably sufficient to maintain health. Vegetable oils and cereals provide the most important dietary source of vitamin E; the content in animal products is low, as it is in seafoods.

DEFICIENCY

Naturally occurring vitamin E deficiency is rare, although it used to be a problem in infants (especially if premature) because the vitamin is transferred across the placenta only in the last few weeks of pregnancy. Human milk is relatively richer in α-tocopherol than cow's milk, but formula feeds are now routinely supplemented with vitamin E. The manifestations of this deficiency are a haemolytic anaemia and thrombocytopaenia. Children with abetalipoproteinaemia are at risk of severe vitamin E deficiency because they lack apolipoprotein B, which is required for the transfer of vitamin E (and other fat soluble vitamins) from enterocytes to the plasma. Untreated, they develop weakness, ataxia and retinopathy with visual impairment. Treatment is with parenteral vitamin E.

EXCESS

The only known adverse effect of a high vitamin E intake is predisposition to bleeding through interference with the metabolism of vitamin K. However, the vitamin has low toxicity and intakes as high as 300 mg per day are generally well tolerated.

Given the importance of the oxidation of low density lipoprotein in atherosclerosis, there has been considerable interest in the notion that supplementation of the diet with antioxidants may protect against this condition but this has not been supported by the results of clinical trials conducted to date, although these are all open to criticism.

ASSESSMENT OF STATUS

Vitamin E can be measured in plasma (normal 25-60 μmol/L) but is better expressed as a ratio to the cholesterol concentration.

Vitamin K

FUNCTION

Vitamin K is a term applied to a group of naphthaquinone derivatives that have an essential role in blood clotting. The natural forms are vitamin K_1 (phylloquinone, phytomenadione) and vitamin K_2 (menaquinone). Vitamin K_3 (menadione) is a synthetic compound and the form used therapeutically. Their structures are shown in Figure 2.16. Reduced vitamin K is a cofactor for the post-translational carboxylation of glutamic acid residues in precursor proteins to form γ-carboxy-glutamate (gla) (Figure 2.17a). Gla has two adjacent carboxyl groups, which enable the protein to bind calcium. This process is catalysed by a carboxylase, and results in the formation of vitamin K epoxide, which is converted back to reduced vitamin K by the successive actions of an epoxide reductase and an NADH-dependent quinone reductase (Figure 2.17b).

Calcium binding is essential to the function of six proteins involved in blood coagulation: factor II (prothrombin), factors VII, IX and XI, and the inhibitory proteins C and S. Calcium facilitates the binding to these proteins of phospholipids that are required for their activity. Inhibitors (e.g. warfarin, Figure 2.16) of the two reductase enzymes involved in the regeneration of reduced vitamin K are used therapeutically as anticoagulants. The efficacy of warfarin treatment is monitored by measurement of the prothrombin time (PT), a measurement of the time that plasma takes to begin to clot after the addition of thromboplastin and calcium. Because of variation between different thromboplastin reagents, it is usual to report the result as a ratio (the International Normalised Ratio, INR) to the PT of control plasma. Therapeutic targets for the INR vary according to the indications for anticoagulation, for example being 2.5 for patients with atrial fibrillation but 3.5 for patients with antiphospholipid syndrome. The INR is also a sensitive test of liver function (see below).

Osteoblasts also contain vitamin K-dependent proteins: osteocalcin, matrix gla protein and protein S. Osteocalcin is the most abundant gla-containing protein in the body and the most abundant protein in bone after collagen. All three have a role in bone mineralisation. However, vitamin K deficiency does not appear to be a cause of defective bone mineralisation. Vitamin K dependent proteins are also present in other tissues involved in calcium metabolism, e.g. the kidneys.

Vitamin K is to some extent synthesised by colonic bacteria and this supplies about half of the body's requirements, about 1 µg/kg body weight/day being an adequate amount in the diet.

DEFICIENCY
Dietary vitamin K deficiency is rare in individuals eating a normal diet because of its widespread availability in vegetables. Deficiency, manifest by a bleeding tendency, can occur in fat malabsorption, e.g. in cholestasis and pancreatic insufficiency. In liver disease, failure of synthesis of clotting factors may cause bleeding even with adequate supplies of vitamin K. When cholestasis, rather than failure of protein synthesis, is the cause of an increased INR, the defect is corrected within 24 h by parenteral administration of vitamin K. In contrast to adults, other-

wise healthy newborn infants are at risk of vitamin K deficiency. Contributory factors to this include poor placental transfer of vitamin K and the initial sterility of the infant's gut, resulting in there being no bacterial vitamin K synthesis; in addition, breast milk is a poor source of the vitamin. It is recommended that babies are given prophylactic parenteral vitamin K shortly after birth to prevent haemorrhagic disease of the newborn. In adults, established deficiency is treated with phytomenadione 10 mg i.v.

In addition to the anticoagulants that target vitamin K, broad spectrum antibiotics may cause transient vitamin K deficiency through an effect on the colonic bacterial flora.

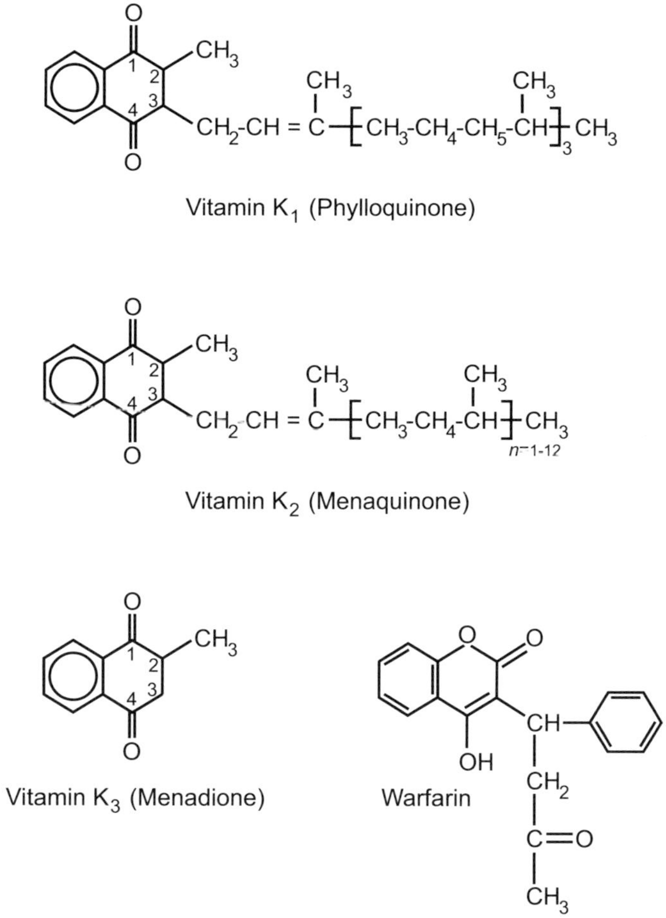

Figure 2.16 Vitamin K and warfarin, a vitamin K antagonist used therapeutically as an anticoagulant

EXCESS
There is no evidence that vitamin K is toxic in man.

ASSESSMENT OF STATUS
Vitamin K status is assessed in the laboratory by measurement of the INR. However, as mentioned above, because prothrombin and the other clotting factors are synthesised in the liver, an increase in the INR can occur in patients with liver disease who are replete in vitamin K. In patients with adequate vitamin K, measurement of the INR provides an excellent indicator of hepatic protein synthetic capacity, and because of the short half life of factor VII, one that responds early to deterioration.

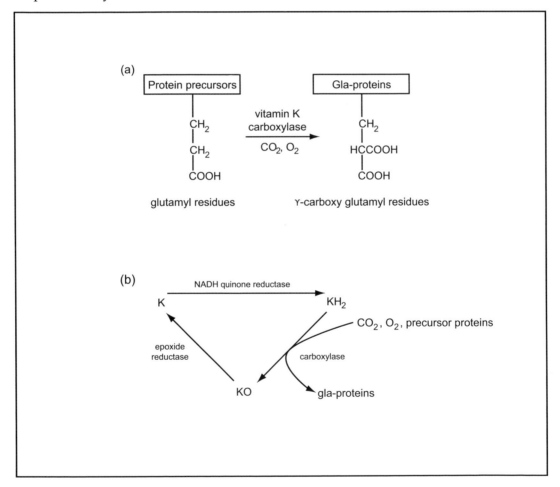

Figure 2.17
a. The γ-carboxylation of glutamate residues in proteins
b. The reactivation of vitamin K

Further reading

Brody T. Nutritional Biochemistry (2nd edition). San Diego, California: Academic Press, 1999.

Frayn K. Metabolic Regulation. A Human Perspective (2nd edition). Oxford: Blackwell Science, 2003.

Geissler C, Powers H. Human Nutrition. Edinburgh: Churchill Livingstone, 2005.

Mann J, Truswell S (eds). Essentials of Human Nutrition (2nd edition). Oxford: Oxford University Press, 2002.

www.food.gov.uk/multimedia/pdfs/nutguideuk.pdf

Chapter 3

Digestion, absorption and malabsorption

Introduction

The digestion of food and the absorption of the nutrients it contains is a complex process that depends on the functional integrity of most of the alimentary tract and its associated organs. Digestion involves mechanical, physical and chemical processes, whereby food is macerated, mixed with enzymes, coenzymes and other substances essential to the processes of digestion and absorption, and transported at an appropriate rate to the regions of the gut where the absorption of nutrients takes place. Absorption involves both energy-dependent and independent mechanisms of varying complexity. During these processes, considerable quantities of fluid (up to 8 L/24 h), minerals, enzymes and other substances are secreted into the gut. The greater bulk of this undergoes reabsorption. At the same time, the alimentary tract provides a route for the excretion of waste products, including indigestible dietary components (e.g. some fibres), bile salts and pigments, and material shed from the lining of the gut. This whole process is orchestrated by interrelated neural and humoral mechanisms. Neural mechanisms include pathways originating in the central nervous system and local pathways that constitute the enteric nervous system; the most important hormones are secreted by the alimentary tract itself.

In essence, digestion begins in the mouth, where food is mixed with saliva (containing amylase) and is macerated by the cutting and grinding action of the teeth (a process that may be compromised in individuals with defective dentition, malocclusion or disease of the oral cavity). Swallowing delivers food to the stomach, where further mechanical and chemical processing occurs. It is then normally released at a controlled rate into the small intestine, where the major parts of both digestion and absorption of nutrients take place. The residue passes into the large intestine, where some further digestion (by colonic microorganisms) takes place and much of the remaining fluid is reabsorbed. Residual material is stored in the distal large bowel prior to excretion. The major functions of the various parts of the alimentary tract are shown in Figure 3.1.

While it has long been recognised that the pancreas and liver have other functions that are not directly related to digestion, the same is also true of the gastrointestinal tract. Of particular importance is its barrier function, which prevents the ingress of potentially harmful material, particularly microorganisms.

Major functions of regions of the alimentary tract and associated organs

Region of alimentary tract	Functions
Oral cavity	Maceration of food Secretion of saliva Secretion of enzymes and initiation of digestion
Oesphagus	Transport
Stomach	Secretion of acid and pepsinogen Further mixing and digestion Controlled delivery of contents to the small intestine Secretion of gastrin Secretion of intrinsic factor Secretion of ghrelin
Duodenum, proximal jejunum	Secretion of various enzymes Further digestion Major site of absorption Secretion of secretin and cholecystokinin
Liver, biliary system	Secretion of bile salts and alkali
Exocrine pancreas	Secretion of enzymes and alkali
Distal small intestine	Absorption of bile salts and vitamin B_{12}
Large intestine	Further digestion (largely by micro-organisms) Absorption of fluid and some nutrients
Rectum	Storage of residue prior to excretion

Figure 3.1 Major functions of regions of the alimentary tract and associated organs related to the digestion of food and the absorption of nutrients

The peri-oral skin is continuous with the epithelium of the gut and the peri-anal skin: effectively, the lumen of the gut is 'outside' the body. Disruption of the integrity of the gut can facilitate invasion of the body by bacteria, with potentially serious consequences. This barrier role of the gut is referred to in more detail in Chapter 5. In addition, the gut contains tissue that is part of the immune system (the mucosa-associated lymphoid tissue, MALT), and is an important endocrine organ. While hormones such as gastrin, secretin and cholecystokinin, which act primarily on the gut itself, were among the earliest hormones to be described, a considerable number of other hormones have since been discovered, some of which are of importance in the regulation of appetite, e.g. ghrelin.

The alimentary tract has a rich blood supply. During the post-absorptive phase, the combined blood flow to the stomach, intestines, pancreas, liver and spleen (not a digestive organ, but sharing the same blood supply) is about 20% of cardiac output, but this increases considerably in the period immediately following a meal. The venous drainage of the stomach and intestines is into the portal venous system, which drains to the liver, providing it with some 70% of its total blood supply. Thus, absorbed nutrients are transported to the liver, where they undergo many metabolic transformations, rather than directly to the systemic circulation. The only major exception is long chain triacylglyerols, which are absorbed into the lymphatic system: the relevance of this is discussed later.

Digestive secretions and gut motility

Oral cavity

Digestion begins in the mouth, where food is macerated by the action of the jaws and tongue (the crushing force exerted by the molars has been shown to exceed 100 Newtons), and is mixed with saliva containing amylase and lubricating mucins. Amylase splits α1-4 links in glucose polymers, i.e. starches, principally amylopectin (branched) and amylose (straight chain). Amylase cannot split the α1-6 links that constitute the branch points in amylopectin nor terminal α1-4 links (see p.24). The products of its action are maltose, maltotriose (dimers and trimers, respectively, of glucose) and α-limit dextrins (polymers containing on average eight glucose residues resulting from the incomplete digestion of amylopectin). Lingual glands secrete a lipase, which begins the process of fat digestion. The secretion of saliva is under neural control; the smell, sight and presence of food in the mouth stimulate the parasympathetic supply to the salivary glands. The submandibular glands secrete approximately 70% of the 1.5 L of saliva secreted each 24 h, most of the remainder coming from the parotid glands.

Stomach

Glands in the wall of the stomach secrete 2-3 L of gastric juice each 24 h: in addition to water, this contains salts, hydrochloric acid, pepsinogens and intrinsic factor. The hydrochloric acid is secreted by parietal cells (also called oxyntic cells). This acid causes some chemical breakdown of proteins, is toxic to many bacteria and activates pepsinogens to produce pepsins (endopeptidases with an optimum pH in the acid range) that cleave peptide bonds adjacent to aromatic amino acid residues. The pepsinogens are secreted by gastric chief (zymogen) cells. A lipase is also secreted into the stomach: unlike pancreatic lipase, it does not require co-lipase as a cofactor. Lingual and gastric lipases account for 20-30% of lipolytic activity in the gut: they allow some digestion of fat to take place even in severe pancreatic insufficiency.

Gastric acid gradually inactivates salivary amylase (though not lingual lipase); it also facilitates the later absorption of calcium and iron (see p.94). The secretion of gastric acid and pepsinogens, and gastric motility, is regulated both neurally (through the vagus nerve and local reflexes) and humorally (principally by gastrin). Cephalic, gastric and intestinal influences are involved in these processes. Thus the sight, smell and taste of food, and the action of chewing, increase secretions in preparation for the delivery of ingested food. The presence of food in the stomach continues this process and is the major stimulus. Some stimulation initially continues when food reaches the duodenum (promoted by gastrin secreted by the duodenal G cells), although secretin, pancreozymin and gastric inhibitory polypeptide inhibit the process.

The hydrogen ions of gastric acid are derived from carbonic acid, which is formed by the hydration of carbon dioxide (Figure 3.2). They are secreted into the lumen of the gut by a H^+,K^+-ATPase. The formation of hydrogen ions also generates bicarbonate ions, which are transported into the interstitial fluid by an antiport that transports chloride ions into the parietal cells. The secretion of gastric acid in response to the ingestion of food can lead to a transient fall in systemic hydrogen ion concentration and the production of an alkaline urine. Acid production causes the stomach to consume more carbon dioxide than is produced by aerobic metabolism so that, unusually, the venous pCO_2 of blood draining from the stomach is lower than that of gastric arterial blood.

The generation of gastric acid does not affect the body's overall hydrogen ion homeostasis, as it is neutralised by bicarbonate secreted into the small intestine. With selective loss of gastric fluid from the body, however, such as may happen during the aspiration of gastric fluid (e.g. because of post-operative ileus) or with vomiting and gastric outflow obstruction, a systemic alkalosis can develop.

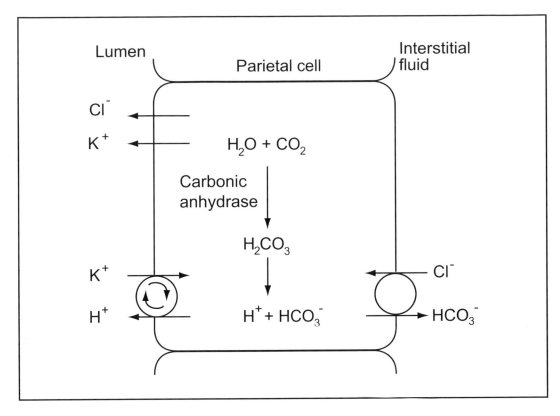

Figure 3.2 The secretion of acid by gastric parietal cells.
The formation of secretory canaliculi is stimulated by the entry of food into the stomach. Hydrogen ions are actively secreted into the gastric lumen against a concentration gradient, in exchange for potassium ions.

The only essential role of the stomach in digestion is the secretion of intrinsic factor, whose sole source is the gastric parietal cells (see p.95). A lack of secretion of intrinsic factor leads to deficiency of vitamin B_{12} even if there is dietary sufficiency. While loss of the other functions of the stomach as a result of disease can compromise digestion and absorption, it does not do so sufficiently to cause the malabsorption syndrome. Malabsorption can, however, be a feature of the Zollinger-Ellison syndrome, a condition characterised by greatly increased secretion of gastrin, and hence gastric acid, which can inactivate pancreatic and small intestinal enzymes.

No significant absorption of nutrients takes place in the stomach, although ethanol can be absorbed to a variable extent, as can certain drugs if they are not ionised at acid pH.

Coordinated contraction and relaxation of the smooth muscle of the stomach effects mixing of food with gastric juice. While the pylorus remains closed, food is held in the stomach. When the pyloric sphincter relaxes, the partly digested food is propelled through the pylorus into the duodenum, the first part of the small intestine. Many factors influence the rate of gastric emptying, including the volume of gastric contents, their chemical nature and osmolality.

The pancreas, liver and small intestine
These organs are responsible for the major part of the digestion and absorption of nutrients; absorption takes place in the small intestine, but is dependent on the production of secretions by all three organs. In the duodenum, food is mixed with bile (containing bile salts, which are essential for fat absorption) and exocrine pancreatic secretions (bicarbonate and various enzymes), together with the secretions of the small intestine itself. The major enzymes are shown in Figure 3.3: many of the proteolytic enzymes are secreted as inactive precursors and are activated only in the lumen of the gut.

The principal digestive enzymes active in the small intestine

Pancreas

Enzyme	Precursor	Activator	Action
carboxypeptidase A and B	procarboxypeptidase A and B	trypsin	exopeptidase
chymotrypsin	chymotrypsinogen	trypsin	endopeptidase
elastase	proelastase	trypsin	endopeptidase
trypsin	trypsinogen	enteropeptidase	endopeptidase
amylase	none	chloride ions	cleaves α1-4 linkages in glucose polysaccharides
colipase	procolipase	trypsin	anchors lipase to mixed micelles
lipase	none	none	hydrolyses triacylglycerols
cholesteryl esterase	none	none	hydrolyses cholesteryl esters

The principal digestive enzymes active in the small intestine (cont.)

Enzyme	Precursor	Activator	Action
phospholipase A	prophospholipase A	trypsin	hydrolyses phospho-lipids
deoxyribonuclease, ribonuclease	none	none	cleaves nucleic acids to form oligo-nucleotides

Intestinal mucosa

Enzymes	Precursor	Activator	Action
aminopeptidases	none	none	cleave N-terminal amino acids from peptides
dipeptidases	none	none	cleave dipeptides to amino acids
enteropeptidases	none	none	activate trypsinogen
α-limit dextrinase*	none	none	converts α-limit dextrins to glucose
maltase	none	none	cleaves maltotriose and maltose to glucose
lactase	none	none	cleaves lactase to glucose and galac-tose
sucrase-isomaltase*	none	none	cleaves sucrose to glucose and fructose
nucleases	none	none	release bases from nucleotides

Figure 3.3 The principal digestive enzymes active in the small intestine. Exopeptidases release terminal amino acids from proteins; endopeptidases cleave internal peptide bonds. The various peptidases are specific for peptide bonds involving particular amino acids.
*each enzyme is a subunit of a single protein

PANCREAS

Approximately 1.5 L of pancreatic juice is produced per 24 h. As with the secretion of gastric juice, cephalic, gastric and intestinal phases of secretion are recognised, the latter being responsible for more than 70% of pancreatic secretion. The cephalic phase is neurally mediated; the gastric phase is mediated both neurally and by gastrin. The intestinal phase is wholly humoral, the major hormones responsible being secretin and cholecystokinin-pancreozymin (CCK-PZ). Secretin (the first chemical agent to which the term 'hormone' was applied, by Bayliss and Starling in 1902) is secreted by cells in the proximal small intestine in response to the presence of acid and peptides. The pancreas responds to secretin by producing large volumes of bicarbonate-rich, enzyme-poor fluid; the alkalinity is required to neutralise gastric acid and provide an optimum pH for the enzymes secreted into the lumen of the small intestine. CCK-PZ is also secreted by proximal small intestinal cells, in response to the presence of peptides, amino acids and long chain (>10 carbon) fatty acids. It has two distinct functions in the gut: it stimulates contraction of the gall bladder, ejecting bile into the duodenum, and stimulates the secretion of pancreatic enzymes. To some extent, both secretin and CCK-PZ also augment each other's primary activity in the pancreas. However, unlike secretin (as far as is known), CCK-PZ is secreted by many other tissues, including the nervous system where it may act as a neurotransmitter.

The process of bicarbonate formation and secretion by the pancreatic exocrine cells is similar to that of acid formation and secretion in the stomach, but in the opposite direction: bicarbonate is secreted into the lumen of the pancreatic ducts while hydrogen ions are pumped into the interstitial fluid. The bicarbonate concentration in pancreatic juice increases with increasing flow rate, from a basal concentration of 20 mmol/L to a maximum of approximately 140 mmol/L.

LIVER

The liver is the source of bile, which is essential for the absorption of dietary fat. The secretion of bile by the liver is determined primarily by the rate of return of bile salts to the liver in the enterohepatic circulation, but the ductal epithelial cells modify this fluid by secreting a watery, bicarbonate-rich fluid. This process is stimulated by secretin, with gastrin and glucagon having minor roles. Up to 1 L of bile is produced each 24 h. Bile is stored in the gall bladder, which contracts under the influence of CCK-PZ, expelling bile through the common bile duct into the duodenum.

The components of bile essential for the absorption of dietary fats are the bile salts (Figure 3.4). These are salts of bile acids, which are derived from cholesterol (for which they represent an important pathway for excretion). The liver synthesises cholic and chenodeoxycholic acids (the primary bile acids); these are converted by intestinal bacteria to deoxycholic and lithocholic acids, respectively. Small amounts of the latter are present in bile via the enterohepatic circulation. The primary bile salts undergo conjugation in the liver with glycine and taurine before they are secreted; this renders them water-soluble and is essential for their function.

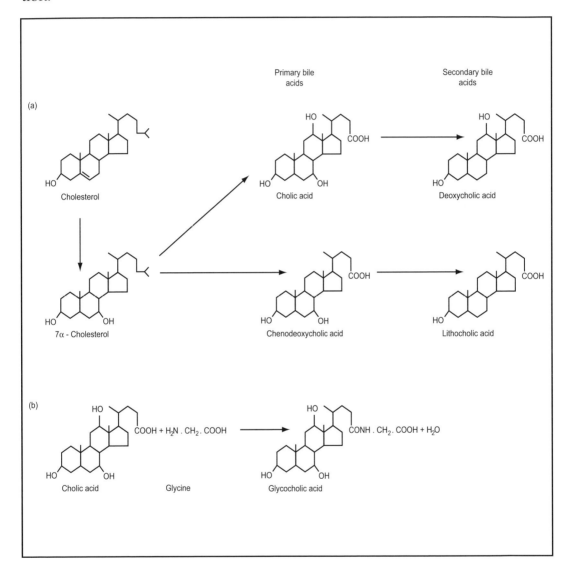

Figure 3.4
a. The structure of bile salts and their formation from cholesterol
b. Conjugation of cholic acid with glycine to form glycocholic acid

Bile salts have two major functions. Since they are amphipathic (i.e. have both hydrophilic and hydrophobic domains), they aid the emulsification of dietary fat prior to its digestion. They can also aggregate to form disc-shaped micelles, in which the hydrophobic domains are projected inwards and the hydrophilic domains project outwards. Lipids enter these micelles, cholesterol being drawn into the hydrophobic centre while phospholipids and mono- and diacylglycerols become orientated with their hydrophobic domains in the interior and their hydrophilic domains on the surface (see Figure 3.5). The formation of these mixed micelles is essential to the process of fat absorption.

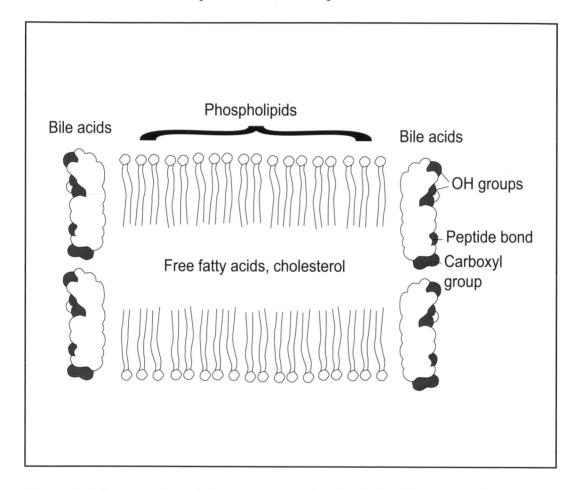

Figure 3.5 Cross sectional diagram of a mixed micelle. These are disc-shaped particles with an outer layer of bile acids and phospholipids enclosing a polar core of fatty acids, monoacylglycerols and cholesterol. At the brush border of enterocytes, the lipids diffuse out of the micelles and enter the cells where their rapid re-esterification maintains a low concentration, thus maintaining a favourable gradient for diffusion

At least 90% of bile salts are reabsorbed (mainly in the terminal ileum) and return to the liver whence they are resecreted. This process is essential to fat absorption: *de novo* synthesis of bile salts is insufficient to supply the amount needed for fat absorption. Thus, although fat absorption takes place in the proximal small intestine, disease of the terminal ileum that reduces the absorption of bile salts can also cause malabsorption of fat, as can bacterial deconjugation of bile salts (see p.102). The bile also contains bile pigments (waste products of bilirubin metabolism) cholesteryl esters and phospholipids. Many xenobiotics, including drugs, are excreted in bile after hepatic conjugation. Although the composition of bile is an important determinant of the risk of formation of gallstones, bile is not accessible for analysis.

SMALL INTESTINE

The small intestine itself is a source of some of the enzymes that are involved in digestion (see Figure 3.3). Of particular importance is enteropeptidase, which is liberated from the brush border membrane by bile salts and activates chymotrypsin, and the disaccharidases (disaccharides themselves are poorly absorbed). These are located in the outer part of the brush border, the membrane of the microvilli on the luminal aspects of the enterocytes (intestinal epithelial cells).

The structure of the small intestine is beautifully suited to its function. The lining is not smooth but consists of villi: finger-like projections 0.5-1.0 mm long, each richly vascularised by capillaries (Figure 3.6). There are 20-40 villi to each square millimetre of mucosa. The apical membrane of individual enterocytes is folded into microvilli, which constitute the brush border across which the absorption of nutrients takes place. These structural features have the effect of greatly increasing (by a factor of several hundred) the absorptive capacity of the small intestine over what would be expected were it to be smooth. Transport across enterocytes occurs at their apical aspects (presented to the lumen of the gut) and their basolateral aspects adjacent to blood capillaries and lymphatic vessels. Enterocytes turn over rapidly. They are formed in the crypts between the villi and migrate up to the tips, whence they are sloughed into the lumen, thus contributing some 30 g protein/24 h to the quantity that has to be digested.

Approximately 1.5 L/24 h of fluid (succus entericus) is secreted into the small intestine from the crypts in a process involving active secretion of chloride and passive movement of sodium and water. Secretion is stimulated by distension of the duodenum, modulated by neural and humoral mechanisms. In the distal jejunum and ileum there is net absorption of fluid of approximately 7 L/24 h.

The contents of the small intestine (chyme) move through its length as a result of peristalsis: coordinated, progressive waves of contraction of its smooth muscle. In addition, alternate contraction and relaxation of short lengths of the intestine mixes the chyme and facilitates its exposure to the absorptive surfaces. These processes are coordinated by intrinsic neural activity, although modified by external influences. At the junction of the small intestine and large intestine, the ileocaecal valve opens when a peristaltic wave increases the pressure in the terminal ileum; if this exceeds the pressure in the proximal large intestine, a portion of ileal chyme is propelled onwards.

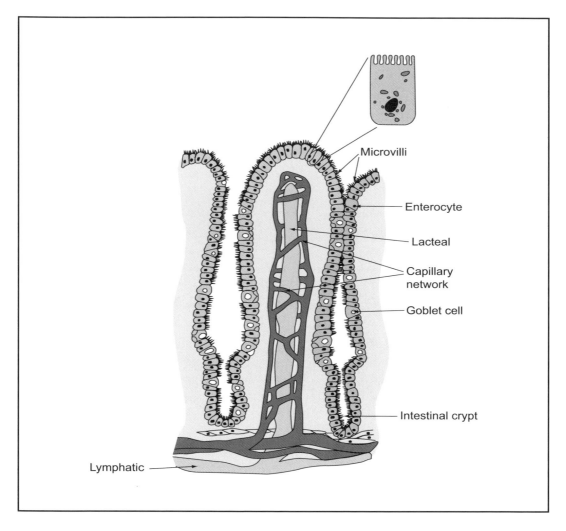

Figure 3.6 Diagram of a vertical section through an intestinal villus; an individual enterocyte is enlarged to show the microvilli, across which absorption takes place.

The large intestine

The major function of the large intestine is the absorption of fluid (approximately 1.5 L/24 h) and salts, and the storage of faeces until they can be voided. While the proximal small intestine is normally sterile and the ileum contains relatively few bacteria, the large intestine has a rich bacterial flora. Some of the body's vitamins, particularly vitamin K, are derived from colonic bacterial synthesis. The bacteria also contribute to digestion through fermentation, producing short chain fatty acids, which are then absorbed. Bacterial fermentation also produces about 500 mL/24 h of gas (flatus) containing hydrogen, methane and hydrogen sulphide among others. Greater volumes are produced if the diet is rich in non-digestible carbohydrates.

As in the small intestine, the large intestine undergoes both mixing and propulsive movements: the latter include slow peristalsis and more vigorous mass movements that propel the faecal material towards the rectum. Rectal distension stimulates the desire to defaecate. Except during mass movements, the contents of the large intestine move slowly. The muscular activity of the large intestine is stimulated by gastric and duodenal distension through local reflexes, modified by hormones and autonomic nervous activity. Various drugs (e.g opiates) decrease the frequency of colonic mass movements.

The digestion and absorption of nutrients

Protein

Intact proteins cannot be absorbed by the gut in human adults, although in the newborn, immunoglobulins present in colostrum can be absorbed without prior digestion. The digestion of proteins involves two groups of enzymes: endopeptidases (pepsins, trypsin, chymotrypsin and elastase) that act on specific interior peptide bonds, and exopeptidases (carboxy- and aminopeptidases) that remove terminal amino acids. The absorption of amino acids is facilitated by transport proteins that act on groups of related amino acids: at least ten have been described. Some, but not all, of the transport proteins cotransport amino acids with sodium. Some di- and tripeptides are also absorbed into enterocytes (utilising a proton-peptide cotransporter), where they are hydrolysed by intracellular peptidases to release their constituent amino acids. The absorption of di- and tripeptides is more rapid than that of amino acids (a matter of considerable relevance to the formulation of products for enteral feeding). Amino acids enter the extracellular fluid by simple and facilitated diffusion. Most absorption of amino acids takes place in the duodenum and jejunum. Food only accounts for about half the total amount of amino acids absorbed, the remainder being derived in roughly equal amounts from digestive juices and desquamated mucosal cells. Less than 5% escapes absorption and passes into the large intestine.

No specific clinical disorder of protein malabsorption has been described (although protein malnutrition is common in many countries). When malabsorption of protein does occur in intestinal disease, other features of malabsorption are invariably present. However, certain intestinal disorders (e.g. Crohn's disease) and NSAIDs (non steroidal anti-inflammatory drugs) can cause protein-losing enteropathy even if absorption is not affected.

Two inherited disorders affect the intestinal absorption of amino acids (and their reabsorption in the proximal convoluted tubules of the kidneys). These are cystinuria (affecting dibasic amino acids) and Hartnup disorder (affecting histidine and other neutral amino acids). There is no deficiency syndrome associated with cystinuria, presumably because the affected amino acids can be absorbed as constituents of di- and tripeptides. Patients with Hartnup disorder may have no adverse effects, but some develop Hartnup disease, the manifestations of which include a pellagra-like rash that is reversed by treatment with nicotinamide. Both decreased intestinal absorption and decreased renal reabsorption are likely to be responsible for this.

Carbohydrate
The digestion of dietary carbohydrates involves the action of amylase (see p.81) in the lumen of the gut to form oligosaccharides. No monomeric glucose is formed because amylase cannot hydrolyse terminal α1-4 links. The oligosaccharides are further digested by enzymes in the brush border to monosaccharides. Glucose and galactose are absorbed together with sodium by a specific transport protein, SGLT-1 (sodium-glucose cotransporter). Inherited deficiency of this receptor is the cause of a severe diarrhoeal disease in infants. Transport of glucose out of enterocytes is by simple and facilitated diffusion utilising the GLUT-2 transporter, which is located on the basolateral membrane. Fructose is absorbed by facilitated diffusion (independently of sodium, utilising the GLUT-5 transporter), and pentoses by simple diffusion.

Although the digestion and absorption of dietary carbohydrate is generally efficient, up to 20% of starch may not be absorbed and passes into the large gut, together with carbohydrates that are resistant to digestion (e.g. celluloses). Here, they become substrates for bacterial fermentation, producing methane, hydrogen and short chain fatty acids.

Carbohydrate is not an essential component of the diet and no specific condition associated with generalised malabsorption of carbohydrate alone has been described (although it may be noted that amylase activity only becomes limiting for carbohydrate digestion when its luminal activity falls below 10% of normal, a level seen only in severe pancreatic insufficiency). Deficiencies of intestinal disaccharidases are discussed later in this chapter.

Fats
The digestion and absorption of fats is a complex process, largely because triacylglycerols (triglycerides), the major dietary fat, are insoluble in water. Malabsorption of fat is usually a feature of the malabsorption syndrome and, for this reason, tests of the integrity of fat absorption have traditionally been used as the basis for tests for malabsorption, although they are now rarely required for this purpose.

The major site of fat digestion is the proximal small intestine. Fats become emulsified into droplets by mechanical action and the detergent action of bile salts and phospholipids (particularly lecithin). Pancreatic lipase preferentially attacks the 1 and 3 bonds in triacylglycerols to produce 2-monoacylglycerols, which also act as detergents. Colipase is essential for this process: it displaces surface bile salts from fat droplets and binds lipase, allowing this enzyme access to the triacylglycerols.

Fatty acids, monoacylglycerols and phospholipids are taken up by bile salt micelles (see p.88) to form mixed micelles. Cholesterol (released from dietary cholesteryl esters by cholesteryl ester hydrolase) and fat soluble vitamins enter the non-polar core of the micelles. The mixed micelles diffuse down their concentration gradient through the unstirred layer (the relatively immobile fluid in immediate contact with the brush border) whereupon the lipids diffuse passively down their concentration gradient into the enterocytes. There is minimal absorption of bile salts in the proximal small intestine: bile salt reabsorption takes place primarily in the terminal ileum, total reabsorption representing 90-95% of the quantity of bile salts secreted in bile.

In the enterocytes, fatty acids and monoacylglycerols with more than 10-12 carbon atoms are re-esterified to form triacylglycerols. These are incorporated with apolipoproteins (principally apolipoprotein B-48) into chylomicrons, which are secreted into the lacteals (intestinal lymphatic vessels) and reach the bloodstream through the thoracic duct. Shorter chain fatty acids pass directly into the blood. Chylomicrons also contain cholesterol, cholesteryl esters and fat soluble vitamins. Some formation of triacylglycerols takes place from acyl CoA (formed from the action of ATP on fatty acids) and α-glycerophosphate (derived from glucose); the latter process is more important during fasting.

Fat digestion and absorption are normally efficient processes, with over 95% of dietary fat being absorbed. Faeces contain about 5% fat, but most of this is derived from colonic bacteria and desquamated cells.

Nucleic acids

Nucleic acids are broken down to nucleotides by pancreatic nucleases; brush border enzymes further metabolise these to phosphate, their sugars (ribose and deoxyribose, both pentoses) and purines and pyrimidines. The absorption of these entities is by passive diffusion.

Water and minerals

Water, sodium and potassium are both secreted and absorbed in the gastro-intestinal tract, but the net process is one of absorption. Water entering the gut includes that ingested as fluids and in solid food, and approximately 8 L of fluid are secreted into the gut per 24 h. In health, only about 200 mL of fluid appear in the stools. Sodium absorption is primarily an active (energy-dependent) process, coupled with the absorption of, for example, glucose and amino acids. Water moves passively along osmotic gradients and potassium moves both by diffusion and by active transport. Potassium secretion in the proximal colon is enhanced through the secretion of aldosterone if potassium intake is high; in the distal colon, active absorption predominates.

Calcium is absorbed by active transport and passive diffusion. Between 30 and 80% of dietary calcium is absorbed, the amount being dependent on the concentration of calcitriol, which stimulates the synthesis of calbindin, a calcium-binding protein, in enterocytes. Calcitriol synthesis, and hence calcium absorption, is stimulated in calcium deficiency. Calcium absorption is inhibited by phosphate, oxalate and phytates (the latter are present in some flours), with which it forms insoluble salts. Calcium can also form insoluble salts with free fatty acids and malabsorption of the latter can decrease the absorption of calcium. Calcium is also secreted into the gut in the various digestive juices. Calcium absorption is never complete (the obligate faecal loss is 2-3 mmol/24 h), so at very low intakes there may be net loss of calcium.

Phosphate absorption is largely passive and increases with increasing dietary intake. Its active absorption is controlled by calcitriol.

Magnesium is absorbed by both passive diffusion and carrier-mediated uptake: to some extent absorption adapts to the body's magnesium requirements and is in part dependent on calcitriol. Unusually, absorption is greater in the ileum than in the jejunum.

Trace elements

Iron absorption is a complex process, which occurs mainly in the duodenum. Ferrous (FeII) iron is more easily absorbed than ferric (FeIII), and organic iron (e.g.

in haem) more easily absorbed than inorganic. Gastric acid secretion is important in iron absorption since the acid reduces the formation of insoluble iron complexes and facilitates its reduction to FeII by ascorbate. Dietary phytates, oxalate and phosphate all reduce iron absorption. The average daily intake of iron in the UK is 20 mg, and although only 5% of this is required to replace obligatory losses in men, more is required in women to replace iron lost in menses and during pregnancy.

Iron deficiency causes anaemia; iron overload is potentially harmful. Iron absorption is facilitated by DMT-1 (divalent metal transporter), an iron-transporting protein expressed on the apical surfaces of enterocytes. Synthesis of this protein is increased in iron deficiency. DMT-1 also appears to have a role in the absorption of other divalent metal ions. Iron transport out of enterocytes at their basolateral surfaces requires the protein ferroportin 1. This transfers the iron to transferrin, which transports iron in plasma. Transferrin concentration increases (and its saturation with iron decreases) in iron deficiency, facilitating the transfer of iron from enterocytes into the bloodstream; when the body is replete in iron, uptake is less and a greater proportion of the iron bound within enterocytes is lost into the lumen of the gut when these cells are shed.

The absorption of elements such as manganese and selenium has not been studied extensively but it appears that, as in the case of iron, absorption is a major factor in their homeostasis. This has major implications for their administration in parenteral nutrition solutions, where the gut is bypassed (see Chapter 5).

Vitamins
The absorption of water soluble vitamins, with the exception of vitamin B_{12}, takes place in the duodenum and jejunum. Active transport, linked to the absorption of sodium, is important for several vitamins (e.g. thiamin, vitamin C), but pyridoxine absorption appears to be by passive diffusion. Dietary folate is present mainly as polyglutamates, which cannot be directly absorbed but must first undergo hydrolysis by brush border enzymes to monoglutamate.

Vitamin B_{12} binds to salivary R protein in the stomach, from which it is released in the duodenum by tryptic activity. It then forms a complex with intrinsic factor (IF), a 45 kDa glycoprotein secreted into the lumen of the gut by the parietal cells of the stomach. The IF-B_{12} complex is absorbed intact by specific receptors on ileal enterocytes, whereupon vitamin B_{12} is released into the bloodstream, where it is transported on a specific binding protein, transcobalamin II.

The fat soluble vitamins (A, D, E and K) are absorbed with other dietary lipids in mixed micelles in the proximal small intestine.

Malabsorption

Introduction

Malabsorption is a failure of the normal absorption of nutrients from the gut despite adequate intake (cf. malnutrition, in which there is inadequate intake). Because the processes of digestion and absorption are so closely linked, there is little to be gained from considering maldigestion and malabsorption as separate processes. Malabsorption can be generalised (affecting a range of nutrients) or affect certain nutrients specifically (particularly lactose in lactase deficiency and vitamin B_{12} in pernicious anaemia).

Malabsorption can be classified on the basis of the level of the defect (e.g. pancreas, liver, intestine), but perhaps more satisfactorily, given the central role of the small intestine, into conditions that affect the processes taking place in the lumen of the gut, disorders of the intestinal mucosa and disorders elsewhere in the small intestine (Figure 3.7).

Conditions causing generalised malabsorption

CONDITIONS AFFECTING PROCESSES WITHIN THE GUT LUMEN

Cause	Mechanisms and comments	Effect
Gastric surgery with bypass Thyrotoxicosis	impaired mixing, intestinal hurry	impaired digestion, reduced time for absorption
Pancreatic insufficiency - chronic pancreatitis - cystic fibrosis - genetic - pancreatic cancer (rarely)	impaired secretion of bicarbonate (so failure to achieve optimum intestinal pH), impaired secretion of digestive enzymes	impaired digestion of fat, protein and carbohydrate
Bile salt insufficiency - cholestatic liver disease - extrahepatic cholestasis - decreased reabsorption of bile salts	decreased availability of bile salts (deconjugation of bile salts with bacterial overgrowth)	malabsorption of fat as a result of failure of formation of mixed micelles

Conditions causing generalised malabsorption (cont.)		

CONDITIONS AFFECTING THE SMALL INTESTINE

Cause	Mechanisms and comments	Effect
Generalised disorders - radiation enteritis - lymphoma	infiltration and destruction of the small intestine	generalised malabsorption
- short gut syndrome	decreased absorptive area	generalised malabsorption
Mucosal disorders - coeliac disease - post-infectious malabsorption (including tropical sprue) - Whipple's disease - Immunodeficiency (congenital and acquired) - Crohn's disease	decreased area for the absorption of nutrients; any acute enteritis can lead to transient lactase deficiency. Crohn's disease affecting the terminal ileum only may lead to depletion of bile salts and failure of absorption of vitamin B_{12}; more extensive disease can affect the duodenum and jejunum	generalised malabsorption

CONDITIONS AFFECTING THE GUT WALL

Cause	Mechanisms and comments	Effect
Intestinal lymphangiectasia	lymphatic obstruction	malabsorption of fat

Figure 3.7 Conditions causing generalised malabsorption

It is beyond the scope of this book to discuss the individual conditions that can cause malabsorption in detail, although some for which laboratory investigations are important in diagnosis are described in the following paragraphs. In the UK, the most frequent cause is coeliac disease although, worldwide, acute and chronic infections (e.g. tropical sprue) are important causes.

Specific causes of malabsorption

COELIAC DISEASE

The basis of this condition is sensitivity to gliadin, a component of gluten, which is present in wheat, barley and rye. It has an incidence of approximately 1 in 1000 in the UK. Genetic and other factors appear to be important in its pathogenesis: the condition can be demonstrated (although is not always symptomatic) in 10-15% of first degree relatives of affected individuals and there is a strong link with the DQ2 antigen of the HLA complex.

Although the condition was described in the first century AD and the clinical features delineated in detail by Samuel Gee in 1888, it was not until the 1940s that the central role of cereals was recognised by Dicke, a Dutch paediatrician. During the winter of 1944-45, there was a famine in the north of The Netherlands, then still occupied by the German Army. Dicke observed that some children's health actually improved during this time, only to relapse after the cereal supply was restored. Dicke and his colleagues subsequently demonstrated that the gluten fraction of wheat flour was responsible for these children's ill health.

Endomysial and tissue transglutaminase antibodies are demonstrable in the great majority of patients with the condition. Transglutaminase is a constituent of endomysium and is the target of a T cell mediated autoimmune response. Transglutaminase acts on gliadin in a way that enhances the response of T cells to gliadin in susceptible individuals. Exposure to gluten results in damage to enterocytes, particularly in the more proximal small intestine. In the most severe cases this leads to the characteristic sub-total villous atrophy that is demonstrable on histological examination of biopsy specimens, accompanied by a chronic inflammatory infiltrate in the lamina propria.

The condition can present at any age from infancy (typically on weaning) to late adulthood. The symptoms are variable in severity, ranging from tiredness and general malaise through to a classic malabsorption syndrome. Endomysial and tissue transglutaminase antibodies (both IgA) are highly sensitive and specific for the condition (approaching 100% for sensitivity and specificity in both cases) and are valuable for screening. IgA anti-gliadin antibodies have sensitivities and specificities of the order of 85%. Anti-reticulin antibodies are frequently present but are less specific. It should be noted that whereas isolated IgA deficiency occurs in about 1 in 500 of the general population, it is seen more frequently in patients with coeliac disease (approximately 2%). When there is a strong suspicion of coeliac disease but tests for IgA endomysial or tissue transglutaminase are negative, the presence of IgG antibodies should be sought; IgG anti-gliadin antibodies may also be detectable. However, the diagnostic sensitivities and specificities for all IgG antibodies are inferior to those for IgA antibodies. The definitive diagnosis is histological, but a typical clinical presentation and positive antibody tests are often regarded as sufficient evidence on which to commence treatment, a response to which confirms the diagnosis. The IgA antibodies become undetectable in blood with successful treatment. Tests for malabsorption are not required.

The condition is treated with a gluten-free diet, which usually brings about a rapid clinical (and histological) improvement, though it is only necessary to repeat the biopsy if the response to treatment is poor. If in doubt, the diagnosis can be confirmed by reintroduction of gluten followed by biopsy to show the typical damage, but in practice this is rarely required. Haematinics should be given initially to replenish body stores.

Even with strict adherence to diet, there is an increased risk of osteoporosis in patients with coeliac disease. There is also an increased risk of both lymphoma (T cell type) and adenocarcinoma of the small intestine; these risks are reduced by treatment with a gluten-free diet. Some patients have the condition in association with dermatitis herpetiformis, a blistering eruption of the skin. This responds to a combination of oral dapsone and a gluten-free diet.

DISACCHARIDASE DEFICIENCY
Deficiency of lactase is common. There is a natural decline in its activity after weaning, and while deficiency is present in 5-15% of adults in northern Europe, it is the norm in some races, with over 70% of adults in South East Asia being affected. However, many individuals with lactase deficiency are asymptomatic because they deliberately avoid milk and dairy products. The severity of symptoms in symptomatic individuals varies considerably: nausea, abdominal distension and cramps, diarrhoea and excessive flatus following milk ingestion are typical.

The diagnosis is usually made on the basis of the symptoms and their relation to (and resolution following exclusion of) milk in the diet. The diagnosis can be confirmed by a lactose tolerance test (a rise in blood glucose concentration of less than 1.1 mmol/L following the ingestion of a 50 g lactose load indicates lactase deficiency) or by measuring the enzyme in a biopsy sample, but this is rarely necessary. An alternative approach is to measure breath hydrogen. The principle is that hydrogen is not produced by mammalian metabolism; hydrogen in exhaled gas is derived from colonic bacteria. An increase in breath hydrogen to above 20 ppm indicates increased bacterial fermentation, such as occurs if undigested lactose is delivered to the colon with its rich bacterial flora. This is a highly sensitive test, but has low specificity: increased breath hydrogen is also seen in intestinal bacterial overgrowth (see p.102). The procedure is performed using a point of care testing apparatus.

In addition to primary lactase deficiency, lactase deficiency can occur secondarily to many other intestinal ailments, including coeliac disease and inflammatory bowel disease. It can also occur in, and may persist transiently after resolution of, gastroenteritis. Congenital deficiencies of sucrase-isomaltase and maltase have been described, but are rare.

PERNICIOUS ANAEMIA

This is an autoimmune disease that prevents the absorption of vitamin B_{12} and leads to a megaloblastic, macrocytic anaemia and neurological damage that classically comprises a peripheral neuropathy and damage to the posterior and lateral columns of the spinal cord (sub-acute combined degeneration). The latter is irreversible if of long standing. Dementia is a late complication.

The condition occurs more frequently in the elderly (1 in 8000 over the age of 60), and in women more frequently than men. There is an association with blood group A and with other 'organ-specific' autoimmune diseases (e.g. vitiligo, hypothyroidism). There is atrophic gastritis with achlorhydria and an increased risk of stomach cancer.

Ninety percent of patients with pernicious anaemia have parietal cell antibodies, although these are not specific to the condition. Antibodies to intrinsic factor (IF) are much more specific but are demonstrable in only about half of people with the condition. These latter antibodies are of two types: one prevents the binding of vitamin B_{12} to IF (blocking antibody), the other (binding antibody) blocks the binding of the IF-B_{12} complex to its receptor.

The diagnosis is based on the demonstration of a macrocytic anaemia with low serum concentrations of vitamin B_{12} in the absence of dietary deficiency (seen only in strict vegetarians), coupled with positive autoantibodies. If the findings are typical, it is often not considered necessary to demonstrate megaloblastic erythropoieisis on a bone marrow smear. The Schilling test (a test of B_{12} absorption, in which the absorption of isotopically labelled vitamin B_{12} with and without intrinsic factor is compared) is no longer available in the UK.

Patients with pernicious anaemia may have mild jaundice (typically a lemon-yellow colour from a combination of jaundice and pallor); this is a result of ineffective erythropoiesis leading to increased formation of bilirubin in the bone marrow.

Treatment is with intramuscular hydroxocobalamin, usually given three monthly after initial repletion of body stores; it must be continued throughout life.

Haematological response to treatment is rapid and can cause hypokalaemia and iron deficiency, such that supplements of potassium and iron may be required.

Other patients who are at risk of vitamin B_{12} deficiency include those who have had total gastrectomies (who are unable to produce intrinsic factor) and those with terminal ileal disease or ileal resection (who are unable to absorb the IF-B_{12} complex). Vitamin B_{12} concentrations should be monitored in such individuals but prophylactic vitamin B_{12} is often given routinely.

PANCREATIC INSUFFICIENCY

Chronic pancreatitis is an uncommon condition, with an incidence in the UK of about 1 in 2000 of the population (though much higher in some tropical countries). It is a progressive inflammatory condition that eventually leads to endocrine and exocrine insufficiency, although these are late complications. The typical (though not invariable) presenting feature is severe, episodic, upper abdominal pain that radiates to the back.

Most cases are associated with calcification: chronic excessive alcohol ingestion is the most frequent cause in the UK but is not implicated in the tropical form. In up to a third of cases no obvious cause can be identified, although an increasing number are being identified as due to genetic mutations, for example of the trypsinogen gene. There are many potential causes of chronic obstructive pancreatitis, which can also lead to pancreatic insufficiency, but this is much less common.

Imaging is the mainstay of the diagnosis of chronic pancreatitis. If present, pancreatic calcification seen on a plain abdominal radiograph is diagnostic. The gold standard investigation is endoscopic retrograde choledochopancreatography (ERCP), but this technique is not without risk. Ultrasonography (increasingly performed endoscopically), spiral computerised tomography and magnetic resonance imaging are also used. It should be noted that these techniques provide morphological diagnoses but do not assess function.

There is no single reliable biochemical test for chronic pancreatitis *per se*. In the past, two types of investigation for pancreatic insufficiency have been used. Direct tests involve intubation of the duodenum (or pancreatic duct) and collection and analysis of secretions for bicarbonate and enzyme activity following stimulation either with a test meal (the Lundh test) or hormones (secretin and pancreozymin or caerulein); indirect tests involve the oral administration of a test substance from which a marker molecule is liberated by pancreatic enzyme activity that is then absorbed and excreted in the urine where it can be measured. The two most widely used test substances were N-benzoyl L-tyrosyl *p*-aminobenzoic acid (NT-

PABA), from which *p*-aminobenzoic acid is released by the action of chymotrypsin, and fluorescein dilaurate, from which fluorescein is liberated by pancreatic esterase (the pancreolauryl test).

The direct tests are superior in terms of both sensitivity and specificity but are demanding on the patient and on medical expertise. They are now rarely performed other than in a research setting. Further information is available for the interested reader in the texts cited in Further Reading at the end of the chapter. The sensitivity of the indirect tests for mild disease (arguably when they could be most useful) is poor (less than 50%) and although they enjoyed a vogue, neither is now used routinely in the UK. Indeed, the tests' materials (a diagnostic kit in the case of the pancreolauryl test) are no longer available in the UK.

The measurement of the activity of pancreatic enzymes in the plasma, so important in the diagnosis of acute pancreatitis, is of no value in chronic pancreatic insufficiency. In this condition, the measurement of enzymes in faeces is helpful in diagnosis: the measurement of faecal elastase is currently the only widely available biochemical test for pancreatic insufficiency and is recommended for this purpose by the British Society of Gastroenterology. Elastase is secreted in pancreatic fluid, is not degraded during its passage through the gut and is stable in faeces *in vitro*. It can be measured using a commercially available immunoassay. A small study showed it to have 63% sensitivity for the diagnosis of mild pancreatic insufficiency, but 100% for moderate and severe insufficiency. It discriminates well between pancreatic and non-pancreatic causes of chronic diarrhoea (defined as the passage of more than 3-4 loose or liquid stools per day and/or a 24 h stool weight of greater than 200 g).

The most important aspect of the treatment of chronic pancreatitis is effective pain control. Pain on eating may itself contribute to poor nutrition in addition to the effects of the pancreatic insufficiency. Maintenance of adequate nutrition is important and pancreatic enzyme supplements may be helpful in achieving this. Patients should be advised to abstain from alcohol and smoking. Surgery may be appropriate if an obstructive cause is identified or to treat intractable pain.

BACTERIAL OVERGROWTH

Overgrowth of bacteria in the small intestine can cause malabsorption by deconjugating bile salts and rendering them inactive. This is most frequently associated with anatomical abnormalities of the gut, which may be iatrogenic (e.g. following surgery, particularly partial gastrectomy with construction of a blind duodenal loop) or acquired (e.g. small intestinal diverticulosis, internal fistulae in Crohn's disease).

Many investigations have been used for the diagnosis of this condition. The definitive technique is probably aspiration and culture of fluid from the small intestine. This has good specificity and sensitivity but requires intubation of the patient. It can give false negative results because of sampling error and is demanding on the bacteriology laboratory. False positive results can also occur: the small intestine is not sterile, and organisms may be detectable that represent colonisation with no clinical sequelae.

The measurement of urinary indicans (bacterial metabolites) is insensitive and should no longer be used. Various breath tests have been described as surrogate markers of bacterial overgrowth. They fall into three categories. The glycocholate breath test involves giving isotopically carbon-labelled (^{13}C or ^{14}C) glycocholate by mouth. Bacterial metabolism of this bile salt releases labelled glycine, giving rise to labelled carbon dioxide, which can be measured in the expired gas. Sensitivity is fair but specificity poor. Better in both respects is a breath test in which the test substance is isotopically labelled xylose. Metabolism of this pentose sugar by bacteria leads to the excretion of labelled carbon dioxide in the expired gas. The third approach is to measure breath hydrogen (see p.99). The performance of this test is improved if an oral dose of glucose is given: this provides a substrate for bacterial action.

The hydrogen breath test has the advantage that it does not require the administration of isotopes (radioactive in the case of ^{14}C) or the provision of the facilities for measuring them. In practice, however, patients are often treated on the basis of a high index of clinical suspicion and the diagnosis confirmed retrospectively by the response to treatment. If it is feasible, surgery to correct the anatomical abnormality should be considered. Prokinetic agents (e.g. octreotide) may be of value. Antibiotics may need to be given long term, but in some instances single or cyclical courses are effective. Appropriate measures should be taken to maintain adequate nutrition.

Clinical features of malabsorption

The clinical features in generalised malabsorption stem from two problems: the effects of deficiency of nutrients, and the effect of non-absorption of nutrients that then pass into the large gut. The classic clinical feature is steatorrhoea, i.e. the passage of bulky, offensively smelly, pale-coloured stools that are difficult to flush away. This is diagnostic of malabsorption when present, but it is only seen in severe cases. Other effects of the passage into the gut of substances that are normally absorbed include abdominal distension, borborygmi and flatulence (a result of bacterial fermentation) and diarrhoea (multifactorial, but in part a result of the cathartic effect of bile salts); however, most chronic diarrhoea is due to causes other than malabsorption. Abdominal pain is uncommon, except in chronic pancreatitis.

Features related to the malabsorption of nutrients may be generalised (e.g. weight loss, general debility, decreased growth velocity in children) or specific (e.g. breathlessness, tiredness and other features of anaemia as a result of haematinic deficiency; easy bruising as a result of vitamin K deficiency; osteomalacia/rickets as a result of malabsorption of vitamin D). Some of the clinical features of malabsorption are summarised in Figure 3.8.

Clinical features of malabsorption	
Clinical feature	**Cause**
Diarrhoea, steatorrhoea, borborygmi, excessive flatus, abdominal distension	Retention of nutrients; bacterial fermentation in large bowel
Weight loss, growth failure	Generalised malabsorption
Abdominal distension	Ascites secondary to hypoalbuminaemia
Anaemia	Impaired absorption of iron (microcytic), and folate and vitamin B_{12} (macrocytic)
Metabolic bone disease	Malabsorption of vitamin D
Easy bruising (uncommon)	Deficiency of vitamin K
Evidence of specific deficiencies	Specific deficiencies

Figure 3.8 Clinical features of malabsorption

Diagnosis

HISTORY AND EXAMINATION
A diagnosis of malabsorption may be suggested by any of the features discussed above, particularly if more than one is present or if features of nutrient deficiency are present together with gastrointestinal symptoms. The appearance of gross steatorrhoea is so characteristic that, if present, it establishes the diagnosis.

In addition to symptoms directly related to malabsorption, features of importance in the history include any family history of coeliac disease or a personal history of overseas travel, excessive alcohol intake, diabetes, abdominal pain, previous gastrointestinal surgery, exposure to radiation or infection with HIV.

Careful clinical examination is mandatory, paying particular attention to the abdomen, and looking for evidence of weight loss and specific nutrient deficiencies. Inspection of growth charts can be informative in children.

SIMPLE INVESTIGATIONS

A list of appropriate simple laboratory investigations is presented in Figure 3.9. If the results of these are all normal, malabsorption is unlikely unless of very recent onset.

It is inappropriate to be dogmatic about the use of more specialised investigations. The widespread availability of endoscopy, allowing direct visualisation of virtually the entire gut (with the exception of the distal ileum) has had a major impact on the use of laboratory investigations. These techniques are now being complemented, and in some cases replaced, by wireless capsule endoscopy, in which the patient swallows a device that allows images of the mucosa of the gut to be captured by an extra-corporeal receiver system, thus obviating the need for endoscopy (though not, as yet, permitting biopsies to be taken).

It is logical to consider the investigation of generalised malabsorption in two stages: first, to establish the diagnosis, second, to establish the cause (although as noted above, the first may be obvious on clinical grounds alone). Although none of the features of generalised malabsorption is specific to any one cause, certain combinations are more suggestive of some conditions than others, and this can be helpful in planning a patient's investigation. Thus the presence of steatorrhoea with a history of excessive alcohol intake is highly suggestive of chronic pancreatitis; poor growth and anaemia in a child is suggestive of cocliac disease, and abdominal distension and diarrhoea following milk ingestion is characteristic of lactase deficiency.

FURTHER INVESTIGATIONS

The use of laboratory investigations for malabsorption has been bedevilled by the multiplicity of investigations, their complexity, a lack of standardisation and varying protocols.

For many years, measurement of faecal fat excretion was regarded as the gold standard investigation for the diagnosis of malabsorption. However, it is unpleasant for all concerned, requires strict adherence to a diet with an adequate fat intake for the period of collection (usually three days) and should now be consigned to the history books. Its passing has spawned numerous other techniques aimed at assessing fat absorption. These fall into two categories: breath tests and direct examination of faeces.

Simple investigations in suspected malabsorption	
Investigation	**Possible abnormality in malabsorption**
Full blood count; serum iron, folate and vitamin B_{12}	Anaemia; evidence of haematinic deficiencies
ESR	Increased in inflammatory conditions
Serum	
urea	Low in protein deficiency
albumin	Hypoalbuminaemia
calcium	Hypocalcaemia (after allowing for low albumin)
phosphate	Hypophosphataemia
alkaline phosphatase	Increased
magnesium	Hypomagnesaemia
C-reactive protein	Increased in inflammatory conditions
thyroid function tests	Evidence of thyrotoxicosis, which can decrease intestinal transit time

Figure 3.9 Simple investigations in suspected malabsorption

In the breath tests, patients ingest a fat meal containing a triacylglycerol tracer labelled with ^{13}C or ^{14}C. Samples of the expired gas are collected and analysed for labelled carbon dioxide. In malabsorption, the amount of label excreted is reduced. The most widely used tracer has been ^{14}C-triolein. Although the results of this test compare well with those of faecal fat measurement, and it can be performed at an outpatient appointment, it requires administration of a radioactive isotope (if a ^{14}C-labelled tracer is used) and facilities for measuring the isotope (mass spectrometry for ^{13}C, scintillation counting for ^{14}C). It is invalid in individuals with conditions in which the metabolism of fats or excretion of carbon dioxide is abnormal, for example, diabetes mellitus and chronic obstructive pulmonary disease. It is therefore rarely used in clinical practice.

In the direct faecal examination tests, a faecal sample is stained for fat and examined under the microscope. Many protocols have been described. The technique described by Fine and Ogmji (see Further Reading), in which both the number and size of fat particles is assessed, is claimed to have comparable specificity and sensitivity to faecal fat measurements but would appear to require considerable expertise to perform properly.

The assessment of faecal fat excretion is a test for generalised malabsorption. Tests involving measurement of the absorption of D-xylose (a pentose) have also been used for many years for this purpose, although they test only absorption (into the enterocytes) and not digestion. D-xylose is absorbed intact from the gut and is little metabolised, so that most of an ingested dose appears in the urine. The test involves giving a test dose of D-xylose by mouth (5 g or 25 g, though the latter can induce an osmotic diarrhoea) and measuring either the plasma concentration of xylose at 1 h after ingestion or the urinary excretion over a period of five hours. The urine test is probably a more sensitive indicator of impaired absorption. However, results are dependent on the rate of gastric emptying, the volume of distribution in the body (increased, for example, in oedematous states) and renal function, and it is an insensitive test for mild degrees of malabsorption. It is now rarely performed. Other marker sugars have been used, and in some cases appear to perform better, but in practice the ready availability of small intestinal biopsy has rendered them obsolete.

Indeed, tests other than those listed in Figure 3.9 are now rarely used to demonstrate that a patient's clinical presentation may be due to malabsorption. Once the diagnosis has been entertained on clinical grounds and support for it provided by the results of one or more of these investigations, the next step is to seek a specific cause. The investigations that are appropriate for this purpose will depend on the clinical presentation and may include measurement of faecal elastase, antibodies to endomysium and tissue transglutaminase, small intestinal biopsy and imaging techniques.

For completeness, it is important to point out that chronic diarrhoea is a common complaint, but is frequently not related to malabsorption. In the absence of evidence of malabsorption, investigations may include, for example, colonoscopy, a search for faecal pathogens and investigations for factitious diarrhoea (e.g. as a result of laxative abuse).

Management
The principles of the management of malabsorption are in theory straightforward: the underlying cause should be treated appropriately and measures taken to ensure that adequate nutrition is restored and maintained. In some instances, e.g. lactase deficiency, this is a simple matter. For some, however, particularly in cases of pancreatic insufficiency, not only is the underlying condition irreversible,

but its effects cannot be entirely ameliorated. When this situation pertains, provision of nutrition support assumes an important aspect of management and this topic is discussed in detail in Chapter 5.

Further reading

Fine KD, Ogmji F. A new method of quantitative fecal fat microscopy and its correlation with chemically measured fecal fat output. Am J Clin Pathol 2000; **113**: 529-534.

Ganong WF. Review of Medical Physiology (21st edition). New York: Lange, 2003.

Högenauer C, Hammer HF. Maldigestion and malabsorption. In: Feldman M, Friedman LS, Sleisenger MH (eds). Sleisenger and Fordtran's Gastrointestinal and Liver Disease (7th edition). Philadelphia: Saunders, 2002, pp 1751-1782.

Thomas PD, Forbes A, Green J, Howdle P, Long R *et al*. Guidelines for the investigation of chronic diarrhoea (Tests for malabsorption, 2nd edition). Gut 2003; **52:** Suppl V: v1-v15. Also available at http://www.bsg.org.uk/chronic_diarr.htm

Chapter 4

Nutritional assessment

Introduction

Nutritional status has been defined as the condition of the body resulting from the intake, absorption and utilisation of food, taking into account factors of pathological significance. Assessment of nutritional status is performed to determine whether patients' nutritional needs are being met, to identify those patients likely to have increased morbidity and mortality without nutrition support and to chart progress with time. The ideal method for nutritional assessment would be sensitive, specific and applicable to all clinical situations. It would also be able to assess nutrition-related risks of morbidity and mortality, and predict whether an individual would benefit from nutrition support. In practice, although a number of techniques exist for nutritional assessment, none is ideal.

Nutritional screening tools

Because of the high incidence of malnutrition, it is recommended that all patients admitted to hospital or care homes, or seen in outpatient departments, are screened for nutritional risk at presentation and, if necessary, referred for detailed nutritional assessment. For inpatients in acute settings, this nutritional screening should be repeated weekly. Various screening tools have been devised and the more accurate the screen, the more complex it tends to become. For example, the Likelihood of Malnutrition Index uses biochemical, haematological, anthropometric and clinical information, which imposes economic and practical limits on its use for routine screening.

Subjective global assessment is a clinical method that uses a combination of information obtained from the patient's symptoms, history and examination findings (Figure 4.1). It is more easily incorporated into routine practice and has been shown to have prognostic value but it requires training and time to be used effectively.

The Malnutrition Universal Screening Tool (MUST) is considerably quicker and easier to apply than subjective global assessment. Four areas are explored: a patient's current condition and whether it is clinically stable, the likelihood of deterioration and whether the underlying disease process will contribute to nutritional insufficiency (Figure 4.2). It can be applied reliably by a variety of health care staff following simple training, but it should be remembered that it is a screening tool rather than a diagnostic test.

Subjective global assessment

A. History
1. Weight change
   Maximum weight _____ wt 1 year ago _____ wt 6 months ago _____ current wt _____

   Overall loss in past 6 months: amount = _____lbs; % loss = _____ (NB: lb = 0.45 kg)
   Change in past 2 weeks: _____ increase, _____ no change, _____ decrease

   Other history: (change in clothing size, loose fitting clothing)
   A = no significant change; B = 5-10% weight loss; C = 10% or more sustained weight loss

2. Dietary intake change (relative to normal)

   Have eating patterns changed over last weeks or months? Has amount of food eaten changed? Are there certain foods they used to eat that they no longer eat? What happens if they try to eat more? How do typical breakfast, lunch, dinner compare with 6 -12 months ago?

   A = no significant change; B = poor but improving or borderline but declining; C = starvation, unable to eat

3. Gastrointestinal symptoms (that have persisted for > 2 weeks)

   A = none; B = some symptoms (nausea, vomiting, diarrhoea, anorexia); C = many symptoms

4. Functional capacity

   A = full capacity; B = mild dysfunction; C = severe dysfunction (duration = _____weeks)

5. Disease and its relation to nutritional requirements

   A = no metabolic demand; B = low/moderate metabolic demand; C = high metabolic demand

B. Physical (for each trait specify: A = normal, B = mild-moderate, C = severe)

   Loss of subcutaneous fat (triceps, chest) _____
   Muscle wasting (quadriceps, deltoids) _____
   Ankle oedema _____
   Sacral oedema _____
   Ascites _____

C. Subjective global assessment rating (select one)

   _____ A = well nourished
   _____ B = moderately (or suspected of being) malnourished
   _____ C = severely malnourished

Figure 4.1 Subjective global assessment.
The clinician uses the scoring sheet to rate individual parameters and on the basis of this assigns an overall subjective classification
Adapted from www.hospitalmedicine.org/geriresource/toolbox/pdfs/subjective_global_assessment.pdf

Malnutrition Universal Screening Tool (MUST)

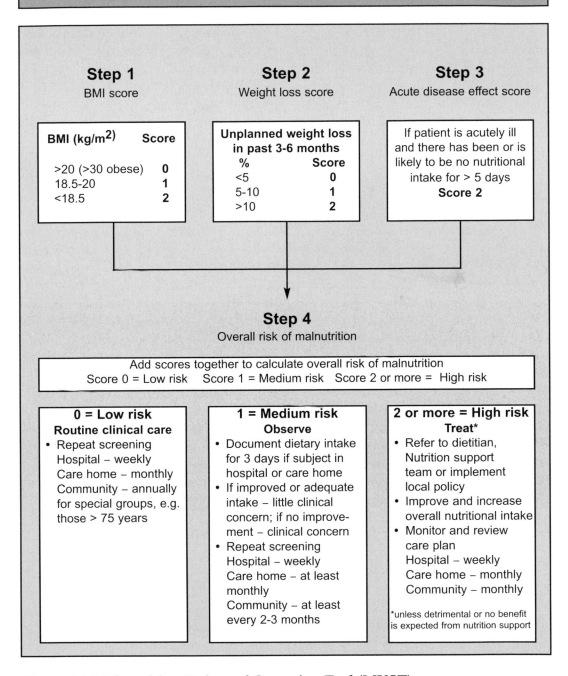

Step 1
BMI score

BMI (kg/m^2)	Score
>20 (>30 obese)	0
18.5-20	1
<18.5	2

Step 2
Weight loss score

Unplanned weight loss in past 3-6 months	
%	Score
<5	0
5-10	1
>10	2

Step 3
Acute disease effect score

If patient is acutely ill and there has been or is likely to be no nutritional intake for > 5 days
Score 2

Step 4
Overall risk of malnutrition

Add scores together to calculate overall risk of malnutrition
Score 0 = Low risk   Score 1 = Medium risk   Score 2 or more = High risk

0 = Low risk
Routine clinical care
- Repeat screening
  Hospital – weekly
  Care home – monthly
  Community – annually
  for special groups, e.g.
  those > 75 years

1 = Medium risk
Observe
- Document dietary intake
  for 3 days if subject in
  hospital or care home
- If improved or adequate
  intake – little clinical
  concern; if no improve-
  ment – clinical concern
- Repeat screening
  Hospital – weekly
  Care home – at least
  monthly
  Community – at least
  every 2-3 months

2 or more = High risk
Treat*
- Refer to dietitian,
  Nutrition support
  team or implement
  local policy
- Improve and increase
  overall nutritional intake
- Monitor and review
  care plan
  Hospital – weekly
  Care home – monthly
  Community – monthly

*unless detrimental or no benefit
is expected from nutrition support

Figure 4.2 Malnutrition Universal Screening Tool (MUST)
Adapted from www.bapen.org.uk/pdfs/Must/MUST-page3.pdf

Dietary assessment

Enquiries about a patient's diet should attempt to reveal any deviation from predicted requirements. Dietary history should include details of intake and any recent changes in eating pattern and should also attempt to identify factors that may contribute to undernutrition. For example, factors contributing to weight loss include loss of appetite as a consequence of illness or drug therapy, difficulties in buying or preparing food secondary to weakness, apathy or musculoskeletal problems, and factors affecting eating, such as poorly fitting dentures or oropharyngeal pain.

Formal methods of dietary assessment are divided into recording current intake, recalling past intake and estimating typical intakes. Recording current dietary intake can be achieved in quantitative or semi-quantitative fashion. A quantitative record requires all food to be weighed or measured prior to being eaten, over a 5-7 day period. This is time consuming and intrusive upon daily life and patients may alter food choices to those that are more easily weighed. A less accurate, alternative method of assessment is for the patient to describe the amount of food eaten to a dietitian, but the ease of this is offset by problems surrounding variations in interpretation of portion size. A photographic atlas of portion sizes can be used to enable greater accuracy. Past intake can be evaluated by asking patients to recall everything consumed in a time period, usually the previous 24 h. While this method rarely provides an adequate dietary assessment when used alone, it can reveal major deficiencies requiring further exploration. This method tends to underestimate energy intake and it is recommended that more than one 24 h period be evaluated for a more representative assessment.

Food frequency questionnaires evaluate customary food consumption over a longer period, patients being asked how frequently they eat foods from different categories. While this approach is useful for population studies, e.g. assessing fruit and vegetable intake in young adults, it is of limited use in the nutritional assessment of individuals. None of these methods of dietary assessment is wholly reliable, and the more rigorous and reliable the method, the more costly it is in terms of time and money.

Clinical assessment

The clinical history and examination are important parts of nutritional assessment. Questioning may reveal evidence of increased nutritional requirements (e.g. because of fever, trauma, burns or sepsis), increased nutrient loss (e.g. through vomiting, fistulae or renal excretion) or decreased absorption (e.g. as a result of diarrhoea, pancreatitis or intestinal resection). Examination may reveal physical signs indicative of generalised nutritional depletion (e.g. muscle wasting or oedema) and specific nutrient deficiency (e.g. anaemia) in addition to those of disease.

Height

Measurement of growth is included as part of the nutritional assessment of children but must be interpreted with regard to the child's genetic background and the relevant reference standards for age and sex. Supine length should be measured using a length board in children less than 18 months; thereafter, standing height can be obtained using an accurately calibrated stadiometer. Correct positioning is essential to ensure reliable measurements. In adults, body height decreases during the day owing to vertebral compression and, ideally, measurements should be made in the morning.

Weight

Body weight and percentage weight loss are readily available indices of nutritional assessment. Scales should be calibrated at regular intervals to ensure accurate results. Sitting scales and weighing beds are available for patients unable to stand, but in practice it may be difficult to ensure that recorded changes reflect only the patient's weight. As body weight reflects total body water, interpretation of changes in body weight may be difficult in hospital patients who have renal, cardiac or hepatic failure with disturbed water homeostasis. Taking measurements of height and weight appears to be easy but in order for the measurements to be accurate they should only be obtained by suitably trained and competent staff.

Body mass index

In people of the same height, variation in weight is mostly due to differences in fat mass. The Quetelet or body mass index (BMI) reflects body fat stores, is a simple method of nutritional assessment and a useful indicator of morbidity and mortality in both patients who are underweight and those who are overweight (Figure 4.3). Adult parameters of BMI are inappropriate in children, whose proportions of body fat vary in an age-dependent manner, and BMI in children should be interpreted by reference to age-specific centiles. Body mass index cannot distinguish between fat mass and lean mass and can be unrepresentative in patients with a large muscle mass, e.g. athletes, in those with wasting disorders or in patients with abnormalities of body weight due to fluid retention from ascites or oedema. It should be noted that a patient who initially has a BMI at the upper end of or above the normal range may lose a considerable amount of weight and still be classified as 'normal'. Cut-off values for defining obesity may be inappropriate in different ethnic groups and alternative cut-off values have been validated for Asians (Figure 4.3).

Body mass index in adults

Body mass index (BMI) = weight (kg) / height ^{2} (m^2)

Caucasians		Asians
<16	severely underweight	
16-18.9	underweight	
19-24.9	normal range	18.5-22.9
25-29.9	overweight	23-27.8
30-39.9	obese	>27.8
≥40	morbidly obese	

Figure 4.3 Body mass index in adults

When direct measurement of height is not possible, e.g. owing to immobility, confusion or spinal disorder, arm demispan or knee height measurements can be used to calculate BMI. Loss of height due to osteoporosis occurs in the elderly and the alternative indices demiquet and mindex have been proposed for use in this age group; these use demispan rather than height (Figure 4.4).

Use of demispan in nutritional assessment

Demispan is measured either:
a)   from the second finger web to the midline chest, or
b)   from the sternal notch in the midline to the tip of the middle finger, both with arms outstretched

Height = (1.2 x demispan in cm) + 71 in males
Height = (1.2 x demispan in cm) + 67 in females

Alternative indices for use in the elderly:

For males > 64 years: demiquet = weight (kg) / demispan (m)^2
For females > 64 years: mindex = weight (kg) / demispan (m)

Figure 4.4 Use of demispan in nutritional assessment

Waist circumference

The distribution of obesity is important in addition to its extent, a central distribution particularly increasing cardiovascular risk. Waist circumference is a simple indicator that has been shown to be of prognostic value with respect to type 2 diabetes and cardiovascular risk; variation suggests that cut-offs appropriate to ethnicity are helpful (Figure 4.5). The waist:hip ratio can also be used to assess abdominal obesity but it is more difficult to measure and yields little extra information.

Waist circumference				
	Increased risk		**Substantially increased risk**	
	Caucasian	Asian	Caucasian	Asian
Male	≥ 94 cm	≥ 78 cm	≥ 102 cm	≥ 90 cm
Female	≥ 80 cm	≥ 72 cm	≥ 88 cm	≥ 80 cm

Figure 4.5 Waist circumference
This is measured midway between the bottom rib and the iliac crest with the patient standing and gently breathing out

Skinfold measurement

Measurement of skinfold thickness, using Harpenden calipers, can be performed to measure subcutaneous fat and the measurements obtained compared with reference values. For an accurate representation, measurement at multiple sites is required (Figure 4.6) but the triceps skinfold (TSF) is that which is most often used. The technique is subject to inter- and intra-observer variation and the mean of three measurements at the site should be used. A change of several kilograms in body weight is required before a change in skinfold thickness is detectable, so the technique is more useful for long-term than short-term assessment. Age and population differences in body fat distribution should be taken into account when interpreting the measurement. Elderly patients and those of Afro-Caribbean origin tend to have a lesser proportion of fat deposited subcutaneously than internally, whilst Asian adults tend to have a greater proportion.

Measurement of skinfold thickness

The skinfold is picked up between thumb and forefinger and the calipers are placed on the skinfold immediately below the fingers. The fingers are then removed and the reading made 2-3 seconds later. Three separate readings should be made and an average taken.

Triceps skinfold: the non-dominant arm is bent to a right angle and a point marked midway between the acromion and olecranon. The skinfold over the triceps is measured at this midpoint with the arm hanging loosely by the side.

Biceps skinfold: over biceps, as above

Subscapular skinfold: just below tip of right scapula

Suprailiac skinfold: just above anterior superior iliac spine in midaxillary line

Figure 4.6 Measurement of skinfold thickness

Mid-arm circumference

Measurement of the mid-arm circumference (MAC), which is the circumference of the non-dominant arm midway between shoulder and elbow, can be used as an indicator of muscle mass (and hence an indicator of protein status) or combined with TSF to estimate muscle protein and fat composition of the upper arm. The values obtained should be interpreted using age and gender-related reference tables. The equations used are as follows (NB: all measurements are made in centimetres):

$$\text{Mid-arm muscle circumference (MAMC)} = \text{MAC} - (\text{TSF} \times \pi)$$

$$\text{Mid-arm muscle area (MAMA)} = \frac{[\text{MAC} - (\text{TSF} \times \pi)]^2}{4\pi}$$

A major advantage of these indices is the accessibility of the upper arm, particularly in immobilised, supine or very sick patients who cannot be weighed. However, the indices do not respond rapidly to changes in nutritional status so are only of value in monitoring longer term trends and are subject to error unless applied correctly.

Functional indices

Assessment of nutritional status by functional indices includes examination of immune status, exercise tolerance and muscle strength.

Total lymphocyte count is the simplest routinely performed measure of immune function; it tends to decrease with malnutrition, correlating with morbidity and mortality. Measurement of delayed cutaneous hypersensitivity has been used for nutritional assessment but it shows low specificity and sensitivity, being affected by illness, e.g. severe bacterial and viral infections, renal failure, haemorrhage, and by drugs such as steroids, immunosuppressants and warfarin.

The measurement of exercise tolerance by ergometer, with concurrent assessment of maximal heart rate, may be useful for nutritional assessment in community settings, although it is dependent on previous exercise tolerance. Reduction in grip strength, measured using a dynamometer, is an index of muscle function. Specificity and sensitivity are improved if sex and age standards are used, but use of the equipment requires cooperation and technique improves with practice. For a more objective measurement, and in patients unable to comply with dynamometry owing to clinical circumstances, electromyography can be performed to assess muscle mass as an indicator of muscle protein.

Summary

Simple tools exist for the assessment of nutritional status and these should be used for regular nutritional screening of all hospital patients and those in long-term care facilities to identify individuals requiring more detailed assessment. A range of more complex methods is available for use in these patients including direct questioning, general examination and specific clinical measurements. All of these methods require a degree of knowledge and skill in order to be used effectively, and none is ideal. Serial measurements to assess trends may be more informative than a basal measurement.

Laboratory investigations

Patients with altered nutritional status often have abnormal biochemistry test results, which has led to the investigation of biochemical parameters as surrogate markers of nutritional status. Plasma protein concentrations have been used as indicators of protein status, examples including albumin, retinol binding protein and transferrin. The half life of the protein reflects the time frame of nutritional change.

Albumin

Albumin is a 67 kDa protein erroneously assumed by many to be a useful indicator of nutritional status. This concept arose because it was assumed that, as albumin has a half life in plasma of about 20 days, a reduced concentration would reflect long-standing malnutrition. However, plasma albumin concentration reflects not only albumin synthesis but also its losses and volume of distribution. The acute phase response tends to decrease plasma albumin concentration, in part owing to inhibition of albumin synthesis by cytokines and its redistribution to the extravascular space.

Albumin concentration can be affected by alterations in hydration status and a decrease of up to 5 g/L can occur on adopting a recumbent posture. In patients with markedly low plasma albumin, the introduction of nutrition support may lead to a further decrease, as the increased intravascular osmotic pressure causes movement of water from the extravascular to the intravascular space.

Albumin is therefore not useful for nutritional assessment, although as its measurement is readily available it tends to be frequently measured and is often misinterpreted. However, it can be indicative of prognosis as it is correlated with disease severity, morbidity and mortality in the critically ill.

Transthyretin

Transthyretin (pre-albumin) is a 55 kDa protein with four identical subunits, which binds with retinol binding protein to form a complex. It is a transport protein for thyroxine. It has a half life of 2.5 days so can be useful as an indicator of short-term response to nutrition support. Transthyretin concentration can be expected to increase by 10 mg/L/24 h if nutrition support is adequate. In some circumstances, e.g. end-stage liver disease and significant inflammation, transthyretin concentrations may decrease and its usefulness is therefore limited.

Retinol binding protein

Retinol binding protein has a molecular weight of 21 kDa and carries retinol bound to transthyretin from the liver to target tissues. It is filtered by the kidneys and degraded in proximal tubular cells. It has a plasma half life of 12 h and responds to short-term changes in energy intake. However, its measurement to assess nutritional status is not valid in vitamin A deficiency and, like transthyretin, its concentration tends to decrease in liver disease and as part of the acute phase response. Retinol binding protein concentrations are affected by renal disease and reference ranges may be influenced by age and gender, making it less attractive for clinical use than transthyretin.

C-reactive protein (CRP)

CRP is the acute phase protein showing the quickest response to injury, increasing after 4-6 hours. Its concentration reflects the catabolic status rather than the nutritional status of the patient, but as catabolism and nitrogen balance are closely linked, CRP can be used in nutritional assessment. The relationship between inflammation and nutritional parameters has resulted in the development of the Prognostic Inflammatory and Nutritional Index (PINI):

$$PINI = \frac{AGP \times CRP}{ALB \times PA}$$

AGP = acid glycoprotein (mg/L), CRP = C-reactive protein (mg/L), ALB = albumin (g/L), PA = pre-albumin (mg/L)

In critically ill patients, a PINI of over 30 has been shown to correlate with the risk of death and the index has found a use as a screening tool for short-term survival.

Insulin-like growth factor I

Insulin-like growth factor I (IGF-I) is produced predominantly in the liver; its plasma concentration is regulated mainly by growth hormone and nutrition. It has a half life of 2-4 hours, is a sensitive marker of acute changes in nutritional status and is a strong predictor of life-threatening complications. It has a wide reference range that is age and gender-related, which complicates interpretation, and it is not used routinely in nutritional assessment.

Fibronectin

Fibronectin is a glycoprotein synthesised in the liver and by fibroblasts, macrophages and endothelial cells, and it has important roles in wound healing, opsonisation and phagocytosis. It has a short half life so has been proposed as a marker of recent changes in nutritional status, its concentration falling after two days of starvation and showing a marked increase by the fifth day of refeeding. However, it has not been shown to be useful as a predictor of clinical outcome.

Transferrin

Transferrin is a 76 kDa protein with two homologous iron-binding domains; it has a plasma half life of 8-10 days. Its function is to bind and transport ferric iron to cell membranes and also to restrict bacterial infection by limiting the availability of free ionised iron required for bacterial growth. Its concentration reflects protein status but not energy intake. Its usefulness in nutritional assessment is limited by the effects of the acute phase response, which tend to decrease the plasma concentration, and iron deficiency, which tends to increase it. Its use to assess nutritional status has been debated but it is no longer considered to be of any practical use.

Other markers

Other markers of nutritional assessment include amino acids and leptin, although neither is currently used as part of routine clinical care. Essential amino acid concentrations in plasma decrease in situations of protein deficiency and those of non-essential amino acids remain normal or rise, resulting in a decrease in the ratio of essential to non-essential amino acids. While this ratio has been considered as a marker of malnutrition, it shows poor sensitivity, is affected by recent food intake and requires complex methods for its measurement. Leptin is a peptide hormone secreted by adipose tissue that, in steady state conditions, acts as a marker for fat stores. It may have a role in nutritional assessment in the future.

Historically, nutritional assessment has involved studies of nitrogen balance and urine creatinine. These techniques are now virtually obsolete but are included here for completeness.

NITROGEN BALANCE

An accurate assessment of nitrogen balance requires calculation of the difference between nitrogen intake and loss and can be used to indicate protein status. Nitrogen input can be gauged from dietary assessment or calculated directly in patients receiving nutrition support. Nitrogen output has traditionally been assessed by measurement of urine nitrogen using the Kjeldahl method or chemi-luminometric techniques; more recently it has been estimated by measuring urine urea excretion.

While nitrogen loss is mainly in the urine, other sources of physiological loss such as hair, skin and faeces can amount to 4 g/24 h. Nitrogen loss from these sites can be increased in the presence of inflammatory processes and significant protein loss can occur from other sources in disease states, for example from burns or fistulae. In addition, there is considerable inter- and intraindividual variation in the amount of nitrogen excreted as urea. Nitrogen balance studies have been considered an important aspect of nutritional assessment in the past. However, due to the potential and summative errors involved in the assessment of nitrogen intake, collection of urine, measurement technique and uncertainty over the contribution of non-urinary nitrogen, these methods are of little practical use.

CREATININE:HEIGHT INDEX

Creatinine is the end product of the metabolism of creatine and creatine phosphate in skeletal muscle. Assuming normal renal function, creatinine excretion rate is an index of creatinine production, which in turn represents the amount of skeletal muscle in the body. Hence, an assessment of muscle mass can be made from urine creatinine excretion, assuming that the 24 h excretion of 1 g (9 mmol) of creatinine is equivalent to 17-20 kg of skeletal muscle. A creatinine:height index can be calculated and compared to reference standards. Although it would appear to be a useful tool, creatinine measurement is influenced by dietary and ethnic factors and there are inherent inaccuracies in prolonged urine collections. Creatinine:height index can give falsely low results in patients with renal failure and in the presence of some medications, for example diuretics, and with the decrease in creatinine clearance that occurs in the elderly, leading to an overestimate of malnutrition.

Summary

Biochemical markers are independent of the size of the individual and can be measured precisely and easily, allowing trends to be monitored. While all these protein markers have been suggested to be useful in nutritional assessment and have theoretical attractions, they all show some disadvantages and hence have not been incorporated into routine clinical practice for this purpose. There is no single laboratory measurement that can be used in isolation in order to assess nutritional status. The main role of laboratory tests is in the confirmation of specific deficiencies, e.g. vitamin B_{12} and iron, and in providing clues to their causes.

Other methods of nutritional assessment

Calorimetry

Energy expenditure is proportional to the amount of metabolically active tissue present in the body, hence it decreases when there is loss of lean body mass. It can either be calculated from the amount of oxygen consumed or from the amount of oxygen consumed and carbon dioxide produced. Direct calorimetry measures heat production by the body; it requires sophisticated equipment and the patient to be placed inside an enclosed chamber, hence it is rarely used in clinical situations. Indirect calorimetry measures oxygen consumption and carbon dioxide production and can be performed at the bedside using small, mobile, open- or closed-circuit units. In the open-circuit units the patient breathes room air and the expired gases are collected for analysis. In closed-circuit methods the patient breathes from an oxygen-containing circuit and, as gas is expired, carbon dioxide is removed. The decrease in gas volumes is proportional to the rate of oxygen consumption and this can be used to calculate the resting energy expenditure (Figure 4.7).

Calorimetry can also provide a measurement of the respiratory quotient (RQ): the ratio of carbon dioxide produced to oxygen consumed. The oxidation of glucose produces an RQ of 1, fat an RQ of 0.7 and protein an RQ of 0.8. An RQ < 0.85 suggests use of endogenous fat stores and hence undernutrition. An RQ > 1 indicates overfeeding and lipogenesis and hence suggests nutritional excess.

Calculation of resting energy expenditure using indirect calorimetry

$$REE\ (kcal/min) = 3.941VO_2 + 1.11VCO_2$$

REE = resting energy expenditure, VO_2 = oxygen consumption (L/min), VCO_2 = carbon dioxide production (L/min)

Figure 4.7 Calculation of resting energy expenditure using indirect calorimetry

Body composition measurement

The measurement of body composition is an important aspect of nutritional assessment both in clinical nutrition and public health. For example, since loss of protein has different significance from loss of fat, measurement of body composition may be more useful than measurement of weight in the assessment of some patients receiving long-term nutrition support. Conversely, assessment of body fat distribution is becoming increasingly important as a marker of cardiovascular risk.

The composition of the body can be considered at five levels of complexity – atomic, molecular, cellular, tissue and whole body. It is possible to measure all 35 of the body's components *in vivo* but not all of the techniques required are applicable outside a laboratory setting. Earliest body composition measurement involved chemical analyses of specific organs and whole cadavers. However, for clinical use, nutritional assessment by body composition measurement involves using either a two compartment model (with the body divided into lean and fat tissue compartments), or a multicompartment model in which the lean tissue compartment is further subdivided (Figure 4.8).

Examples of two compartment models include underwater weighing and isotope dilution. Three compartment models can be constructed in which the fat free mass (FFM) is further subdivided into two: water and the remainder (comprising predominantly protein and minerals). Four compartment models require accurate measurement of total body water and of protein and mineral contents. The densities of protein and mineral can be assumed, but their masses need to be measured using techniques such as neutron activation analysis for body protein and dual-energy X-ray absorptiometry (DEXA) for bone mineral content. Four compartment models that avoid the use of underwater weighing consider the FFM in terms of body cell mass, extracellular water and extracellular solids. Body cell mass can be calculated from measurement of whole body potassium, extracellular water from isotope dilution methods and extracellular solids from bone mineral content, using DEXA. Models of increasing complexity can be constructed using additional independent measurements. However, measurement of body composition using these techniques has not been shown to predict clinical outcomes.

Methods of body composition analysis	
Two compartment models	**Multi-compartment models**
Bioelectrical impedance	Dual-energy X-ray absorptivity (DEXA)
Densitometry	Computerised tomography (CT)
Isotope dilution	Magnetic resonance imaging (MRI)

Figure 4.8 Methods of body composition analysis

MEASUREMENT OF BODY DENSITY

Although it is only a two compartment model, measurement of body density by underwater weighing is considered to be the gold standard owing to its extensive validation. It is based on the principle that an individual's loss of weight underwater is equivalent to the volume of water that his body displaces, which in turn is equivalent to his body volume. The subject is weighed in air, then immersed in water and reweighed. A correction is made for the residual lung volume. The density of the individual may then be calculated as his mass divided by his volume. These parameters enable calculation of percentage body fat, for example from the Siri equation (Figure 4.9). Since the density of the FFM is known to be 1.1 g/mL and that of fat is 0.9 g/mL, if the total body density is known, the percentage of body fat can be calculated from the equation.

More recently, air displacement systems have been developed in which the subject sits in an air-filled chamber instead of under water, e.g. the Bod Pod® (Figure 4.10). This system has two adjacent chambers separated by a diaphragm. The subject is placed in one chamber and the other serves as a reference. Body volume is calculated from changes in pressure based on Boyle's Law.

The Siri equation for the estimation of percentage body fat

D = body density (determined from underwater weighing)
A = proportion of lean body tissue (i.e. the fat free mass)
B = proportion of fat tissue
a = density of lean body tissue (1.1 g/mL)
b = density of fat tissue (0.9 g/mL)

Body density is given by the following equation:
D = (A + B) / [(A/a) + (B/b)]

Given that A = 1 - B, the equation can be solved for B such that:
B = [(1/D) x 4.95] - 4.5

Hence the % body fat = (495/D) - 450

Figure 4.9 The Siri equation for the estimation of percentage body fat

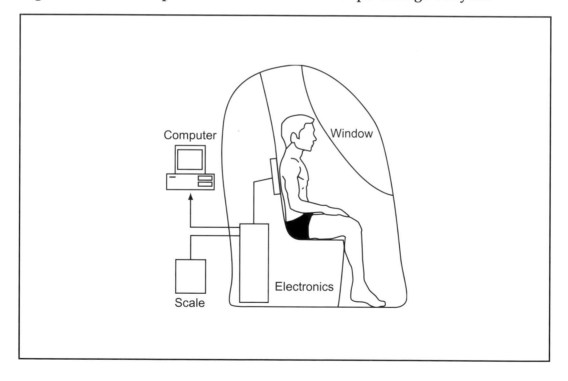

Figure 4.10 The Bod Pod® for measurement of body density by air displacement

ISOTOPE DILUTION METHODS

Isotope dilution methods are based on the principle that the volume of a body compartment can be defined as the ratio of the dose of a tracer to its concentration in that compartment shortly after its administration. A fluid sample is taken to determine a baseline, a tracer such as tritiated water, D_2O or $H_2^{18}O$ is administered and a further sample taken. The method of analysis is chosen according to the tracer used, e.g. scintillation counting for tritium, mass spectroscopy for ^{18}O oxygen and infrared absorption, gas chromatography or mass spectroscopy for deuterium. Water constitutes about 73% of the FFM, hence measured dilution volumes can be used to predict FFM and fat mass (equal to the body weight minus the FFM).

BIOIMPEDANCE ANALYSIS

Aqueous tissues are the major conductors of an electrical current within the body. This fact has led to the use of electrical methods for measuring total body water (TBW) and FFM. Equipment for bioimpedance analysis is available that is suitable for use in clinical settings. The measurements are made by attaching electrodes to the patient's arms and legs. A single, weak, alternating current is passed and the voltage drop from the outer to inner electrodes is recorded to derive the impedance. This value can be used in prediction equations to derive body composition data.

This method of nutritional analysis has the advantage of being quick and relatively easy to perform; the equipment is also reasonably cheap and can be transported to most clinical settings. The accuracy and reproducibility of bioimpedance analysis is dependent on many variables, although some of these can be controlled, e.g. ensuring the measurement is made at least four hours after the last meal. Measurements made in this way tend to overestimate TBW in lean subjects and underestimate it in the obese. Significant errors may occur in patients with known abnormalities of fluid or electrolyte balance, thus limiting its usefulness. However, with these caveats, it is beginning to be used for nutritional assessment in clinical as well as research settings.

WHOLE BODY COUNTING AND NEUTRON ACTIVATION ANALYSIS

Various elements including potassium, nitrogen, calcium and sodium can be measured by a group of techniques involving whole body counting and neutron activation analysis. Measurement of the γ-ray decay of naturally occurring ^{40}K can be used to determine total body potassium, which can then be used as a marker for total body cell mass. However, using conversion factors derived from work on cadavers, it can also be used to estimate FFM. Counting is technically demanding, requiring a good quality detection system and a mechanism to shield the subject and detector from background radiation. Gamma-neutron activation analysis can be used to measure total body nitrogen to calculate total body protein, calcium to determine bone mineral mass and sodium to determine extracellular water. While loss of total body potassium has been shown to be a predictor of poor outcome, measurements are limited to research settings owing to the specialist nature of these methods.

MAGNETIC RESONANCE IMAGING

Magnetic resonance imaging (MRI) involves placing the body in a strong magnetic field, which causes nuclei containing an uneven number of nuclear particles to attempt to align themselves with or against the magnetic field. Only a small proportion of nuclei do become aligned but, on removal of the field, they release energy, the intensity of which can be used to measure the number of hydrogen nuclei in the tissue. The contrast between fat and lean tissues may be enhanced by the use of T1 weighted scans. T1 is the relaxation time taken for nuclei to release their energy and return to random positions; T1 for protons in water is longer than for protons in fat. Abdominal images produced in this way allow separation of subcutaneous adipose and visceral adipose tissue and hence have the potential to monitor change in individual compartments. The wide-spread availability of MRI makes it a possible method for clinical use in the near future, although this would have significant cost implications.

DUAL-ENERGY X-RAY ABSORPTIOMETRY

When an X-ray beam is placed on one side of an object, the intensity of the beam detected on the opposite side of the object is related to its chemical composition, thickness and density. Images are obtained using the attenuation of tissues exposed to X-rays at two peak energies. While DEXA is primarily used to estimate bone mass, it can be used in addition for determination of lean tissue and fat masses. Although it involves X-rays, scan times are short and the dose is low, making it potentially useful for clinical investigations.

COMPUTERISED TOMOGRAPHY

Computerised tomography (CT) is also a measurement technique based on X-rays but it requires the source and detector to rotate in a perpendicular plane around the patient. The anatomical image is similar to that obtained from MRI. However, it can provide more information about the true density of a tissue at each pixel, e.g. bone can be identified as cortical or trabecular on the basis of its density. The major disadvantage of this technique is the radiation exposure involved, which makes it unsuitable for serial measurements.

Conclusion

Assessment of nutritional status is an essential part of clinical care in order to identify patients who would benefit from nutrition support. There is no 'gold standard' for nutritional assessment, but in the majority of patients subjective global assessment, coupled with an objective measurement such as BMI, can provide a reliable assessment. More sophisticated methods have potential for clinical use but have not yet been incorporated into routine practice.

For the future, the advent of microarray analysis brings the prospect of studying individual variation in the metabolism of dietary components. This could result in the ability to provide personalised nutritional assessment and nutrition support.

Further reading

Bates CJ, Nelson M, Ulijaszek SJ. Nutritional assessment methods. In: Geissler C, Powers H. Human Nutrition. Edinburgh: Churchill Livingstone, 2005, pp 573-96.

Gibson RS. Principles of Nutritional Assessment (2nd edition). Oxford: Oxford University Press, 2005.

Thomas B (Ed). Manual of Dietetic Practice (3rd edition). Oxford: Blackwell Publishing Ltd, 2001.

Chapter 5

Nutrition support

Introduction

The prevalence of undernutrition amongst hospital inpatients has been shown to be as high as 40% and recent studies suggest that this figure has changed little since the problem was first quantified some fifty years ago. The effect of under-nutrition on clinical outcome depends on the patient's age, initial body weight and the underlying disease, but even in young, previously fit patients (e.g. admitted following trauma) it is associated with increased morbidity and mortality and prolonged hospital stay (Figure 5.1).

Complications associated with malnutrition in hospital inpatients	
Effect of malnutrition	**Complication**
Impaired immune response	Infection
Decreased respiratory muscle strength	Increased incidence of chest infection
Impaired wound healing	Prolonged recovery
Inactivity	Thromboembolism, pressure sores
Decreased skeletal muscle strength	Fatigue, inactivity, falls
Impaired thermoregulation	Hypothermia

Figure 5.1 Complications associated with malnutrition in hospital inpatients

It is essential that patients who are undernourished, or at risk of becoming under-nourished, are identified and referred for further assessment so that nutrition support that may potentially have a favourable effect on clinical outcome can be instituted. Even obese patients with a history of rapid weight loss may benefit from nutrition support, particularly if their hospitalisation is expected to involve a prolonged period without adequate food intake.

In its simplest form, nutrition support involves the provision of a meal appro-priate for the patient's diet, taste and culture, served in an atmosphere conducive to eating, with assistance from hospital personnel to ensure that it can be consumed. For patients who cannot meet their needs in this way, for example due to increased requirements or decreased appetite, food enrichment can be achieved by the use of high energy substrates or proprietary supplements.

Food enrichment

Nutritional intake can be increased through food enrichment, for example by the addition of butter to potatoes, grated cheese and cream to soups, and jam to puddings. Where this is unsuitable, a range of supplements is available, the contents and flavours differing between manufacturers (Figure 5.2). Modular supplements usually contain just one macronutrient and are typically supplied in powder form. They are useful for patients who require additional protein or energy but whose ability to take food orally is not impaired. Carbohydrate powders can be added to drinks and puddings; protein powders, after mixing with water, can be incorporated into foods such as soup and mashed potato. Fortified puddings can provide additional protein and energy in a small volume, although brands of supermarket desserts often provide a more popular alternative. Nutritionally complete supplements are supplied in cans or cartons containing 200-300 mL; the majority provide about 200 kcal, 10 g protein and contain vitamins and minerals. Supplements of this type are milky in consistency but most are lactose-free. Fruit-based fortified supplements are not nutritionally complete but may be more acceptable to patients. Both types are more palatable when served chilled, although some of the savoury varieties can be heated. It should be noted that bacterial contamination may occur if supplements are left open for prolonged periods. Achieving adequate nutrition using food enrichment and supplements requires the cooperation of the patient and can be time consuming for attendants: it may fail if this time is not available.

Food supplements
Modular supplements: carbohydrate   protein Fortified puddings Fortified supplements (juice type) Nutritionally complete supplements (milky type)

Figure 5.2 Food supplements

Patients whose intake remains suboptimal with oral supplementation by these means require further support by either enteral (gastrointestinal) or parenteral (intravenous) routes. Such support is also required for patients who cannot tolerate oral feeding, including patients with swallowing disorders and those with intestinal failure. Nutrition support should be considered for patients with:

- a body mass index (BMI) of less than 18.5 kg/m^2
- unintentional weight loss of more than 10% in the previous 3-6 months
- little input for 5 days and anticipated poor input for at least a further 5 days
- poor absorptive capacity with high nutrient losses or increased nutrient needs.

The introduction of nutrition support may not always be appropriate and decisions regarding its introduction or withdrawal may occasionally be difficult. Each case should be considered individually with regard to the patient's wishes and with input from all those involved in their care. For patients in a terminal phase of their illness, it may be appropriate to administer nutrition support to relieve symptoms rather than to prolong life. For other patients, complex ethical and legal factors may be involved, and in extreme cases guidance may need to be sought from the Courts.

Nutritional requirements

For appropriate nutrition support, nutrient provision should be matched to the patient's requirements based on their basal metabolic rate (BMR) and any additional needs arising from their current metabolic state.

Energy requirements

There are various methods for calculating energy requirements. Calorimetry (see Chapter 4) is accurate but not easy to use in a clinical setting; the following calculations are practical alternatives.

ESTIMATION FROM BODY WEIGHT

Energy requirements may be calculated from body weight, assuming a requirement of between 25 and 35 kcal/kg/24 h; the higher values are suitable for patients with stresses such as pyrexia and burns.

PREDICTION EQUATIONS

The Schofield equation provides an estimate of basal metabolic rate (BMR) based on weight, age and sex. It can be used with the Elia nomogram (see Further Reading), which allows adjustment for stress to predict energy expenditure in different clinical situations (Figure 5.3).

Schofield equation		
Age (years)	Male BMR (kcal/day)	Female BMR (kcal/day)
15-18	17.6W + 656	13.3W + 690
19-30	15.0W + 690	14.8W + 485
31-60	11.4W + 870	8.1W + 842
>60	11.7W + 585	9.0W + 656

Figure 5.3 Schofield equation for estimation of basal metabolic rate from body weight (W = body weight in kg)

The Harris-Benedict equation (Figure 5.4) estimates basal energy expenditure, which is assumed to be equivalent to the BMR (although this assumption causes a slight overestimate of the true BMR). A stress factor of between 1 and 1.5 should be included to reflect individual circumstances, which adds a degree of subjectivity to the calculation.

Harris-Benedict equation
Male basal energy expenditure = 66.5 + (13.8W) + (5H) - (6.8A) kcal/24 h
Female basal energy expenditure = 655 + (9.6W) + (1.8H) - (4.7A) kcal/24 h

Figure 5.4 Harris-Benedict equation for estimation of basal energy expenditure (W = weight in kg, H = height in cm, A = age in years)

It is important to note that these formulae were derived from studies in healthy subjects. Other prediction equations, for example the Ireton-Jones formula for use in patients in intensive care units, have been derived from work in specific patient groups.

Protein requirements

As protein is the only macronutrient containing nitrogen, protein requirements are sometimes estimated in terms of nitrogen. Approximately 16% of protein is nitrogen, so it is possible to convert an estimate in grams of nitrogen to grams of protein by multiplying by a factor of 6.25. The average healthy adult requires a protein intake of about 0.75 g/kg/24 h, but for hospitalised patients the requirement is likely to be increased to 1 g/kg/24 h (0.15 g nitrogen), increasing further to 1.5 g/kg/24 h in those with sepsis or after trauma. Intercurrent problems such as renal or liver dysfunction with decreased protein handling may prevent the administration of actual requirements as nutrition support.

The estimation of protein requirements from urinary nitrogen is discussed briefly in Chapter 4 but, due to its inherent inaccuracies, it is not generally useful. The protein content of parenteral nutrition tends to be expressed in grams of nitrogen and the energy it provides excluded from the calculated energy content of the feed. This convention may help to ensure that adequate energy is provided by carbohydrate and fat and so help to ensure protein sparing.

Fluid and electrolyte requirements
The basic fluid requirement for an individual is about 30-35 mL/kg/24 h. A positive fluid balance should be expected to account for insensible losses from the respiratory tract and skin and additional losses via these routes should be included when estimating fluid requirements, e.g. 2-2.5 mL/kg/24 h should be provided for every 1°C temperature rise above 37°C. Other sources of fluid loss that can be quantified, if crudely, include vomit, diarrhoea, fistula and drain losses.

An average adult's sodium requirement is ~1 mmol/kg/24 h, assuming normal fluid balance and renal status. Since sodium is lost in the sweat, 15 mmol sodium should be added to each 100 mL additional fluid given to compensate for fluid lost as sweat in the presence of pyrexia. Large fluid losses from the gastrointestinal tract should be expected to lead to a sodium loss of approximately 130-150 mmol/L.

While the basic requirement for potassium is ~1 mmol/kg/24 h, this may be increased to as much as 7 mmol/kg/24 h when refeeding the severely malnourished (see p.151). The potassium content of gastrointestinal fluid loss is much lower than that of sodium (being approximately 5-10 mmol/L), and excess loss is more commonly from the renal tract, for example on recovery from acute tubular necrosis or secondary to the use of drugs such as diuretics or aminoglycosides.

Phosphate requirements may be hard to meet, particularly in the early stages of refeeding, due to rapid cellular uptake (see p.151). The phosphate content of nutrition support preparations is limited by proprietary and stability constraints.

Enteral feeding

When nutrients are delivered to the gut they stimulate the release of gut hormones that help to maintain its integrity. With the exception of most lipids, which are absorbed into the lymphatic system, nutrients are absorbed from the gut into the portal circulation. Enteral nutrition (EN), in which nutrients reach the bloodstream via the gut, is thus more physiological than parenteral nutrition (PN) in which nutrients are delivered directly into the systemic circulation, and has advantages with regard to the maintenance of intestinal integrity. The efficiency of the tight junctions between intestinal cells is, in part, energy dependent, the major metabolic fuel being glutamine obtained from local absorption. The nature of the gastrointestinal microflora affects the local epithelial permeability and is less perturbed by EN than PN. Cytokine concentrations and secretory IgA production are more favourable in patients being fed enterally, rendering the intestinal epithelium less liable to breaching by pathogenic organisms. Enteral nutrition is also cheaper than PN, although not proven to be safer, and so is indicated in patients with a functioning and accessible gut. Indications for EN are shown in Figure 5.5; the only absolute contraindication is mechanical obstruction.

Indications for enteral nutrition

Indication	Example
Disturbed swallowing	Motor neurone disease
Upper gastrointestinal obstruction	Oesophageal stricture
Inability to eat	Head injury, critical illness
Gastrointestinal disease	Pancreatic insufficiency
High requirements	Burns, trauma
Loss of appetite	Anorexia nervosa, cardiac cachexia, cancer
Transition from parenteral nutrition	

Figure 5.5 Indications for enteral nutrition

Route of enteral feeding

The majority of patients requiring enteral feeding receive it through a nasogastric tube. However, there are other routes of administration, determined by the indication for feeding, treatment plan and patient preference. Feed can be delivered directly into the stomach (gastric feeding) or beyond the stomach into the duodenum or jejunum (post-pyloric feeding). The feeding tube can be passed into or beyond the stomach from the nose (or mouth) or directly into the gut (enterostomy) (Figure 5.6). When feeding is predicted to be needed for more than 30 days an enterostomy is likely to be required.

Routes of delivery of enteral tube feeds	
Into the stomach	**Beyond the stomach**
Nasogastric or orogastric tube	Nasoduodenal tube
Gastrostomy	Jejunostomy
Oesophagostomy	

Figure 5.6 Routes of delivery of enteral tube feeds

Nasogastric feeding tubes are usually fine bore 6-9 FG (French gauge – the external circumference of the tube in millimetres) and are inserted with the aid of an integral guide wire. A feeding gastrostomy is a tract between the stomach and abdominal surface used for intragastric feeding, the most common being a percutaneous endoscopic gastrostomy (PEG), which can be performed using local anaesthesia. The placing of a PEG is usually performed by either 'pull through' or 'push' (Seldinger) techniques, or by direct puncture, the first being the simplest and most frequently used. Using the 'pull through' technique (Figure 5.7), an endoscope is passed and the stomach inflated with air. Aided by the endoscope, the anterior gastric wall is punctured with a cannula and a thread or guide wire passed through it into the stomach (a). The thread is retrieved by the endoscopist (b) and the feeding tube is then drawn down into the stomach as the thread is pulled (c).

Gastrostomies can also be placed under fluoroscopic guidance (FPG), a technique that is particularly useful in patients with ascites or those receiving peritoneal dialysis, circumstances that are relative contraindications for PEG feeding. Gastrostomy feeding is used extensively in hospital and in the community for patients who require long-term nutrition support, for example those unable to eat due to neurological disease or those with high requirements such as patients with cystic fibrosis. Skin level gastrostomies have been developed; these are often referred to as buttons. They are particularly useful for children and outpatients who require gastrostomy feeding, owing to their cosmetic advantages and the decreased chance of displacement compared with standard tubes.

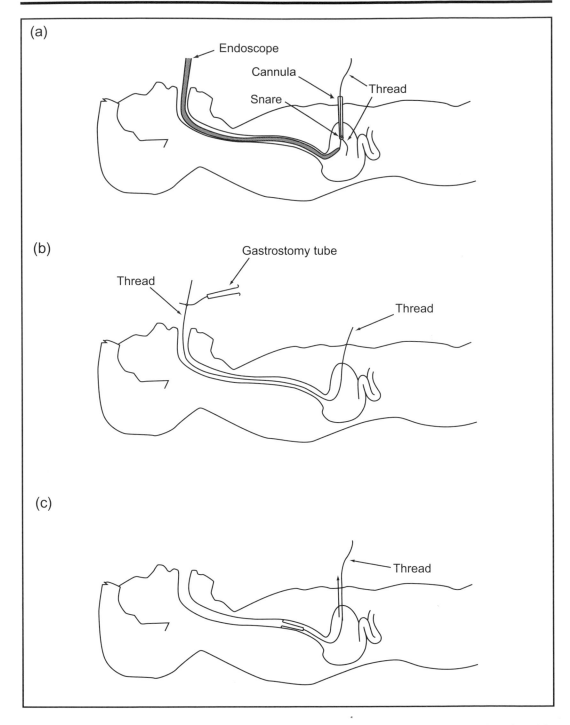

Figure 5.7 Placement of percutaneous endoscopic gastrostomy tube (PEG). Details of the operator's end of the endoscope have been omitted for simplicity.

Nasoduodenal or nasojejunal feeding tubes are used for patients at high risk of pulmonary aspiration and in patients with pancreatitis in whom feeding beyond the opening of the pancreatic duct is considered necessary. Previously, these tubes were placed by endoscopy or fluoroscopy but newer tubes with coiled ends can now be placed into the stomach directly and are self-propelled to the small intestine. The placing of a feeding jejunostomy is most often carried out as an additional procedure in patients undergoing major upper abdominal surgery, when the need for enteral nutrition support is anticipated pre-operatively. The most common technique is that of needle catheter jejunostomy, in which a thin tube is passed through a tunnel in the seromuscular space of the intestinal wall before entering the intestinal lumen.

Composition of enteral feed
In the developing world, puréed, strained food is sometimes administered through nasogastric tubes, although it would not be suitable for jejunal feeding. This practice is associated with a high incidence of tube blockage and feed contamination and in developed countries it is more usual to use commercially prepared feeds. These may be polymeric, disease-specific or elemental feeds.

Polymeric feeds contain whole protein as the nitrogen source and so require a functioning gut for their absorption. Commercial feeds contain vitamins and trace elements and most of them provide 50 g protein/L and 1 kcal/mL. Feeds that contain fibre are also available. In acute illness, their advantage may be to provide short chain fatty acids that have a trophic effect on mucosa. As fibre has potential protective effects, such feeds may be appropriate in patients receiving long-term enteral nutrition.

Disease-specific feeds are formulated with the requirements of particular groups of patients in mind. High energy feeds with 1.2 and 2 kcal/mL can be useful for patients with restricted fluid intakes or high energy requirements. Feeds suitable for patients with chronic renal failure have decreased sodium, potassium and phosphate contents but increased amounts of water soluble vitamins to compensate for losses caused by dialysis. Feeds designed for patients with pulmonary disease provide a greater proportion of energy from fat so that less carbon dioxide is produced during metabolism.

Elemental feeds contain nitrogen as free amino acids or oligopeptides that can be absorbed without prior intraluminal hydrolysis. Their use is indicated in patients with severe impairment of digestion and absorption.

Delivery of enteral feed

Enteral feeds can be administered by bolus or delivered continuously using a pump. A bolus feeding regimen involves the administration of 100-300 mL of feed at intervals during the day at a rate of about 10 mL/min. It tends to be associated with a lower incidence of diarrhoea and may be useful in patients with a tendency to remove feeding tubes. Continuous feeding can usefully be done overnight to supplement suboptimal oral intake during the day. It ensures a continuous carbo-hydrate supply and may facilitate glycaemic control. Intermittent continuous feeding with a daily 'rest period' of more than four hours can utilise the natural protective effect of gastric acidity, as the pH will drop between feeds. A period when the patient can be disconnected from the pump may also increase mobility and self-esteem.

Complications of enteral feeding

Complications of enteral feeding are shown in Figure 5.8. Malposition of the feeding tube can result in pneumothorax or its siting in the trachea or even, occa-sionally, intracranially. It is essential that the position of the tube is checked prior to use by X-ray or by checking that aspirate is acidic by using pH paper. Tube blockage is most commonly caused by using the tube to deliver drugs or by inad-equate flushing of the tube. Drug absorbance may be interrupted or altered during tube feeding. This may be a result of the drug's binding to the tubing or forming an insoluble compound with a component of the feed.

Local physical discomfort due to the presence of a tube is common; rarely, it may cause nasopharyngeal or oesophageal bleeding. Local complications specific to enterostomy tubes include wound dehiscence, infection, leakage and bleeding.

Diarrhoea is common in patients receiving enteral feeds, particularly in those who are critically ill. It is more usually attributable to concurrent administration of antibiotics or non-absorbable carbohydrates (such as sorbitol in medications) than to the enteral feed, particularly in patients with critical illness.

Aspiration of stomach contents into the lungs, causing asphyxia or pneumonitis, is common, particularly in patients with a decreased gag reflex. When feeding is commenced, the feeding tube should be aspirated four-hourly with a syringe and the residual volume noted. A volume of more than 200 mL is associated with an increased risk of pulmonary aspiration. The risk of aspiration is decreased by nursing patients with the bed head elevated by at least 30°. Prokinetic agents, such as metoclopramide and erythromycin, may be used to stimulate gastric emptying and decrease the risk of aspiration. Alternatively, a post-pyloric tube can be placed.

Enteral feeds can become contaminated by bacteria but this is preventable by careful nursing technique during their administration. Particular care should be taken in patients with achlorhydria, who lack the protection of bactericidal gastric acid, and in those who are immunosuppressed. Biochemical complications can occur in patients receiving EN (see later), but these are less common than in patients receiving PN.

Complications of enteral feeding

Type of complication	Example
Mechanical	Malposition Blockage Local physical damage
Gastrointestinal	Diarrhoea Constipation Abdominal distension
Biochemical	Electrolyte disturbances Elevated liver enzymes
Miscellaneous	Pulmonary aspiration Drug-nutrient interactions Contamination of feed Infection

Figure 5.8 Complications of enteral feeding

Parenteral nutrition

In patients whose gut is not functioning, nutrition support can be provided by the parenteral route in which nutrients are delivered into the blood using a venous catheter. As techniques for initiating enteral feeding have improved and its benefits demonstrated, the indications for parenteral nutrition have diminished and it should be reserved for patients in whom enteral intake is inadequate or unsafe and in whom the gastrointestinal tract is non-functional, perforated or inaccessible. Examples of the common reasons for administration of PN in hospitalised patients are shown in Figure 5.9.

Indications for parenteral nutrition

Intestinal blockage

Mechanical obstruction

Paralytic ileus

Pseudo-obstruction

Shortening of bowel

Massive resection

Fistulae

Inflammation

Inflammatory bowel disease

Chemotherapy

Radiotherapy

Other reasons, e.g. multi-organ failure, intra-abdominal sepsis

Figure 5.9 Indications for parenteral nutrition

Parenteral nutrition has been shown to be delivered most effectively by a multi-disciplinary nutrition support team. Such an approach results in both a decreased incidence of complications and in cost savings. Members of the team should include a clinician, nutrition specialist nurse, dietitian, pharmacist and a clinical biochemist. The clinician has overall responsibility for the care of the patients and liaises with other clinical teams involved in their care. The dietitian is involved in the initial nutritional assessment and referral of patients for nutrition support and, within the team, has a role in determining nutritional requirements. The pharmacist is in charge of the manufacture of PN and advises on the stability of proposed regimens and potential drug-nutrient interactions. The specialist nurse is involved in education and communication at ward level with a particular role in advising on the use of intravenous catheters in the administration of PN. The clinical biochemist has responsibility for coordinating and interpreting laboratory investigations and using them to make recommendations for the composition of feeds. This is particularly important with regard to electrolytes and the monitoring of micronutrients. The need for a multidisciplinary approach to oversee all aspects of food provision and nutrition support within hospitals has resulted in the extension of the role of the PN team in some settings.

It is often difficult to predict for how long PN will be required at the point when it is instituted. The majority of patients receive PN for fewer than two weeks although for some it may be lifelong. When the clinical indication for PN has resolved, oral or enteral feeding should be gradually reintroduced and PN decreased accordingly; it should be stopped when it is supplying less than half of the patient's energy requirements. Parenteral nutrition is usually referred to as total parenteral nutrition (TPN) but it can be useful as an addition to enteral intake, for example in some patients who retain limited gastrointestinal function. Once stable, such patients may successfully receive home PN with regular, but infrequent, laboratory monitoring. If PN is administered on a cyclical basis for only part of the day, patients are able to continue the activities of daily living relatively uninterrupted.

Route of administration

Parenteral nutrition can be administered via catheters placed into central or peripheral veins. Central venous catheters are used most often to deliver PN, their insertion requiring placement of the tip of the catheter into the jugular vein or superior vena cava. The insertion and use of central venous catheters carries a risk of morbidity and even mortality, with sepsis being the major complication (Figure 5.10).

Complications of central venous catheters
Air embolism
Arterial puncture
Blockage
Dysrhythmias
Malposition
Nerve injury
Pneumothorax
Sepsis
Thrombosis

Figure 5.10 Complications of central venous catheters

The risk of catheter-related infection is associated with the method and site of insertion, the type of catheter used and the experience of the operator. Ideally, the catheter should be specifically for PN, but in sick patients this may not be achievable. When multilumen lines are used, a dedicated lumen should be reserved for PN. The infection rate is greater with catheters inserted into the internal jugular than the subclavian vein and is so high when the femoral vein is used that this route is not recommended for this purpose. In order to reduce the risk of infection, catheters should be inserted using strict aseptic technique and PN should be set up with the same precautions. Catheter care and dressing should be performed regularly, with gauze dressings being changed every 48-72 h, or when wet, and transparent dressings changed weekly. The line tubing should be changed every 24 h. If an infection is suspected, e.g. from evidence of pyrexia or leucocytosis, feeding through the catheter should be temporarily discontinued and cultures taken from the peripheral blood and from blood taken through the catheter. If infection is proven, appropriate antibiotics should be administered and the catheter may need to be removed. *Staphylococcus epidermidis* and *Staphylococcus aureus*, microorganisms from the patient's own skin, are the most common causes of infection, but infection with Gram negative bacteria, yeasts or fungi can occur, particularly in patients who are immunosuppressed or receiving long-term PN. When PN is to be administered for more than a month, a tunnelled line is preferable; a short segment of catheter is 'tunnelled' under the skin to exit at a distance from the point of entry to the vein. This acts to decrease the incidence of infection.

By placing catheters in a peripheral vein it is possible to avoid many of the risks associated with the use of central catheters, but there is a greater risk of thrombophlebitis. The risk can be decreased by ensuring that the osmolality of the feed is less than 600 mmol/kg, but this imposes constraints on its composition and requires a volume for its formulation that may exceed that allowed in fluid-restricted patients. Other measures that are effective in decreasing the risk of thrombophlebitis associated with peripheral feeding include the use of strict aseptic technique for the insertion of the catheter, rotation of the entry site every 48 h and the use of glyceryl trinitrate patches placed distal to the site of infusion. This route should be considered in patients who are likely to require only short-term PN and do not require central access for other reasons.

Peripherally inserted central catheters (PICCs) are a recent development in the administration of PN. Although the catheter is inserted peripherally, its tip lies in a central vein. Whatever the route chosen for delivery, PN must be administered using an alarmed volumetric pump and the use of a 1.2 μm filter is also recommended to decrease the likelihood of bacterial contamination and to remove particulate matter.

Composition of parenteral feed

Parenteral nutrition needs to contain carbohydrate, nitrogen, fat, minerals, vitamins, trace elements and water and is usually delivered in a single 'all-in-one' bag, although the regimens prescribed for infants may be unstable unless the lipid component is infused separately. The composition of the feed should meet the patient's needs. Various commercially produced solutions are available and for the majority of patients one of these can be selected and minor additions made according to specific requirements (Figure 5.11). For patients with complex requirements, PN solutions can be compounded individually if the hospital's pharmacy is equipped with a suitable sterile production facility. It must be ensured that any prescribed regimen is stable or irreversible lipid/water phase separation ('cracking') may occur. The infusion of cracked emulsions puts the recipient at risk of potentially fatal lipid emboli. The concentrations of electrolytes, particularly divalent and trivalent cations, affect surface charges and hence increase lipid aggregation and the likelihood of cracking occurring.

Content of a typical parenteral feed for an adult male		
Nitrogen	14	g
Glucose	250	g
Fat	100	g
Sodium	80	mmol
Potassium	60	mmol
Calcium	5	mmol
Magnesium	10	mmol
Phosphate	25	mmol
Vitamins and trace elements		
Total energy (non-nitrogen)	2000	kcal
Total volume	2500	mL

Figure 5.11 Content of a typical parenteral feed for an adult male

CARBOHYDRATE

The carbohydrate component of PN is provided by glucose, which is the major monosaccharide in the carbohydrate of a conventional diet. The maximal rate at which glucose can be oxidised is 5 mg/kg/min, which corresponds to 25 kcal/kg/24 h. Infusion at a higher rate than this results in hyperglycaemia, excessive carbon dioxide production and deposition of fat in the liver. Glucose utilisation may be impaired in patients who are sufficiently ill to require PN, particularly the elderly and those with sepsis, and concurrent insulin therapy may be required to prevent hyperglycaemia. Insulin will almost always be required in patients with diabetes mellitus or impaired glucose tolerance who require PN. Other carbohydrate sources that have been used in the past, such as fructose and sorbitol, can precipitate lactic acidosis and are no longer used for PN. Glycerol has been developed as a commercial energy source, marketed as a short-term post-operative feeding preparation, but it is not used as a substrate for PN.

LIPID

The use of fat, which is an efficient source of calories, as an energy source for PN in addition to glucose, circumvents the problems of excess glucose and provides essential fatty acids. Commercially available lipid for PN has traditionally been manufactured from soybean or safflower oils containing long chain triacyl-glyerols, over three quarters of which are made up of essential fatty acids. The mean lipid droplet size is 300 nm, within the range of dimensions of endogenous chylomicrons. Within the circulation, both the lipid component of PN and chylomicrons are cleared by lipoprotein lipase. Lipid can accumulate in the retic-uloendothelial system, impairing its ability to remove bacteria and endotoxins and increasing susceptibility to infection and so should not be infused at rates greater than 0.11 g/kg/h (1 kcal/kg/h). The relatively large amount of polyun-saturated fatty acids and small amount of α-tocopherol contained can result in production of an unbalanced eicosanoid profile and increased lipid peroxidation. This has led manufacturers to develop alternative lipid substrates.

Medium chain triacylglycerols are rapidly taken up by peripheral tissues and oxidised; their metabolism does not require carnitine. Medium chain triacylglyc-erols neither promote eicosanoid synthesis nor provide precursors for oxygen free radicals. However, they are not suitable as a sole lipid source as they do not include essential fatty acids and have a tendency to cause metabolic acidosis. There has been recent interest in the use of structured triacylglycerols as a lipid substrate for PN. These are synthesised by inter-esterifying medium and long chain fatty acids to create mixed triacylglycerol molecules. Lipid preparations based on olive oil can be used to decrease the intake of polyunsaturated fatty acids. Omega 3 fatty acids (fish oils) are being developed for use in PN and may have beneficial effects on eicosanoid and cytokine production and on splanchnic perfusion.

PROTEIN

The nitrogen component of PN is supplied as a mixture of L-amino acids, with essential amino acids providing about 40% of the total amino acid nitrogen. Enrichment with other amino acids may be helpful in particular circumstances and formulations for infants contain additional histidine and tyrosine – amino acids that are considered essential for them. Parenteral nutrition solutions enriched with the branched chain amino acids leucine, isoleucine and valine have been proposed to be beneficial for use in patients with hepatic encephalopathy, in order to correct the altered ratio of branched chain to aromatic amino acids, but although they may reduce the progression of encephalopathy, they do not reverse it.

Glutamine comprises more than 60% of the skeletal muscle free amino acid pool and 20% of the plasma free amino acid pool. It is an important precursor for nucleotide synthesis and a substrate for rapidly dividing cells, such as those of the immune system and intestinal mucosa. Although not an essential amino acid, glutamine may become so during metabolic stress. There is evidence to suggest that the use of parenteral glutamine improves the outcome of patients after critical illness. Glutathione is a tripeptide composed of cysteine, glutamine and glycine, which has antioxidant activities. Its addition to PN may attenuate cell destruction by oxygen free radicals. Arginine is important in nitrogen metabolism but has a particular role in the generation of nitric oxide and the addition of arginine to PN may prove to be a way of manipulating nitric oxide formation. Carnitine is a trimethylamine comprising lysine, methionine and glycine residues and is important in fatty acid oxidation as it facilitates fatty acid transport across mitochondrial membranes. It may prove a useful addition to PN formulations, particularly in infants and young children whose capacity to synthesise and store carnitine is poorly developed.

ELECTROLYTES

The electrolyte content of a typical bag of PN is shown in Figure 5.11. Sodium is usually given in the form of sodium chloride. Potassium is given as a combination of about two thirds potassium acetate and one third potassium phosphate. Acetate is useful in correcting acidosis resulting from diarrhoea or urinary bicarbonate loss and can be given as the sodium salt if required. Calcium is usually added as calcium gluconate and magnesium in the form of magnesium sulphate.

VITAMINS AND TRACE ELEMENTS

Early studies establishing micronutrient requirements related to enteral nutrition only, and the control of absorption of some vitamins and trace elements is exercised at the level of the gut. The development of long-term PN, with micronutrient provision based on enteral requirements, led to recognition of clinical deficiencies of some micronutrients, from which their parenteral requirements were defined.

Once compounded, the vitamins within PN solutions may be subject to degradation, e.g. vitamins A and E by light. The solutions should be protected from light during administration and this is usually achieved by placing the bag inside a light-shielding cover. Vitamins and trace elements can be obtained as commercially available mixtures that meet recommended daily intakes for micronutrients by the parenteral route (Figure 5.12). Those for administration to children have proportions to suit the requirements of that age group. Nevertheless, further supplements may be appropriate in special circumstances, e.g. additional thiamin in starved patients, when the body's thiamin reserves would be expected to be relatively low.

In the USA, but not the UK, vitamin preparations do not contain vitamin K, to avoid possible interaction with oral anticoagulants. Vitamin K is contained in the lipid component of PN, and although probably not present in a greater amount than in a normal diet, a note of the potential for interaction of PN with oral anti-coagulants should be made in the patient's records.

Monitoring of patients receiving parenteral nutrition

In order for their response to be observed and to prevent the development of complications, patients receiving PN should be monitored by both bedside and laboratory assessment. Assessment should include evaluation of the patient's gastrointestinal function, for example the presence of nausea, vomiting, diarrhoea or fistula output, whether bowel sounds are present and the nature and volume of any gastric aspirates. Actual nutrient intake should be recorded and patients weighed twice weekly.

At the bedside, the patient's state of hydration should be evaluated by clinical examination and by assessment of fluid balance charts, taking into account any fluid in addition to that contained in the feed and output other than urine, e.g. vomit, diarrhoea, sweat and loss from drains. In patients receiving PN, blood glucose concentration should be measured every four hours at the bedside; once stable, daily urinalysis for glucose is adequate. Patients receiving EN should have daily urinalysis at the start of feeding.

At the time that nutrition support is commenced, laboratory testing is often being performed frequently for the management of the underlying illness. Laboratory markers can be used as part of nutritional assessment (see Chapter 4) and so have a potential role in the selection and monitoring of patients receiving nutrition support. However, the majority of these markers, for example transferrin and retinol binding protein, are influenced by the acute phase response, limiting their usefulness in patients commencing PN, who are often critically ill. Patients fed enterally retain the homeostatic functions of the gut, so such intensive monitoring is not usually necessary.

Recommended daily intakes of micronutrients by the parenteral route

Trace elements

	µmol	mg
Iron	20	1.1
Zinc	38-100	2.5-6.4
Copper	8-24	0.5-1.5
Iodine	1.0	0.127
Manganese	3-15	0.15-0.8
Fluoride	50	0.95
Chromium	0.2-0.3	0.01-0.015
Selenium	0.4	0.03
Molybdenum	0.2	0.02

Vitamins

Retinol	1000	µg
	3300	IU
Ergocalciferol	5	µg
	200	IU
Tocopherol	10	mg
Vitamin K	150	µg
Ascorbic acid	100	mg
Thiamin	3.0	mg
Riboflavin	3.6	mg
Pyridoxine	4.0	mg
Niacin	40	mg
Vitamin B_{12}	5.0	µg
Panthothenic acid	15	mg
Biotin	60	µg
Folic acid	400	µg

Figure 5.12 Recommended daily intakes of micronutrients by the parenteral route

Plasma sodium, potassium, calcium, phosphate and magnesium concentrations should be measured prior to commencing PN, and liver and renal function should be assessed, as abnormalities may require prescription of a bespoke feed rather than a standard prescription, e.g. with additional phosphate in hypophos-phataemia or restriction of potassium in renal failure. Triglyceride concentrations should be measured prior to commencing PN and at intervals afterwards and, if raised, the lipid content of the feed should be reduced.

Zinc, copper and selenium may be measured prior to the introduction of PN, particularly if prolonged feeding is anticipated. Plasma zinc concentration correlates with that of plasma albumin; although low values are associated with zinc deficiency, they may not always reflect total body zinc concentration but instead are a reflection of the acute phase response. Plasma copper is related to the concentration of the copper binding protein caeruloplasmin, which increases during the acute phase response and hence may mask copper deficiency. Other micronutrients, except for iron (via measurement of haemoglobin, ferritin or transferrin) and folate, are not usually assessed by laboratory testing unless a specific deficiency is suspected.

A scheme for the laboratory monitoring of patients receiving PN is shown in Figure 5.13; if specific abnormalities occur, more frequent monitoring may be needed until they are corrected.

Concentrations of manganese should be measured every 3-6 months, and those of aluminium annually, in patients on long-term parenteral therapy to assess potential toxicity. Patients on long-term PN can become deficient in vitamins, particularly in vitamin B_{12} if there is a history of gastric or ileal surgery, and in fat soluble vitamins in those with malabsorption or liver disease; measurement of plasma concentrations, directly or indirectly, may allow detection of deficiencies and enable replacement. Monitoring of patients on long-term PN should also include intermittent gall bladder ultrasound for evidence of cholelithiasis and echocardiography for evidence of thrombosis around the central venous catheter.

Complications of parenteral nutrition
Patients receiving PN should be monitored to assess their response, to prevent the development of complications (Figure 5.14) and to determine their suitability for transfer to enteral feeding. Clinical biochemists have an important role in anticipating and preventing complications, and lessening their severity if they do occur.

Monitoring of nutrition support

Parameter	Frequency
Sodium, potassium, urea, creatinine	Baseline Daily until stable Then 1-2 times a week
Magnesium, phosphate	Baseline Daily if at risk of refeeding syndrome Then 3 times a week until stable Then weekly
Calcium, albumin	Baseline Then weekly
Liver function testing (including INR)	Baseline 2 times a week until stable Then weekly
Glucose	Baseline 1-2 times a day (at least) until stable Then weekly
Zinc, copper	Baseline 2-4 weekly depending on results
Selenium	Baseline if at risk of depletion Further testing dependent on baseline
C-reactive protein	Baseline Then 2-3 times a week
Full blood count	Baseline 1-2 times a week
Iron, ferritin	Baseline Then every 2-4 weeks
Folate, vitamin B_{12}	Baseline Then every 2-4 weeks
Manganese	Every 3-6 months (home PN)
Vitamin D	Every 3-6 months (long-term support)
Bone densitometry	On starting home PN Then every 2 years

Figure 5.13 Monitoring of nutrition support

Metabolic complications of parenteral nutrition
Hyper/hypoglycaemia
Hyper/hypokalaemia
Hypomagnesaemia
Hypophosphataemia
Hyper/hyponatraemia
Refeeding syndrome
Hyper/hypocalcaemia
Hypertriglyceridaemia
Hepatic damage
Metabolic bone disease
Micronutrient deficiency or toxicity

Figure 5.14 Metabolic complications of parenteral nutrition

DISTURBANCES OF GLUCOSE HOMEOSTASIS

Hyperglycaemia occurs relatively frequently in patients receiving PN, particularly in the elderly and those who have sepsis or pre-existing glucose intolerance. It should be treated using continuous intravenous infusion of insulin from a syringe pump, striving for strict glycaemic control to optimise benefit from PN. Rebound hypoglycaemia can occur after abrupt cessation of PN both when insulin is being used concurrently and when it is not. However, in the latter case it is very uncommon now that lipid-containing admixtures are used.

DISTURBANCES OF ELECTROLYTE BALANCE

Disturbances of electrolytes can occur, particularly if pathophysiological changes are not anticipated at the time that a patient's feed is prepared. Hyperkalaemia is particularly likely in patients with renal failure or metabolic acidosis. Hypokalaemia tends to occur when replacement does not take account of excessive losses, e.g. from the gastrointestinal or renal tracts, or in patients who become anabolic following a catabolic phase. Hyperchloraemic metabolic acidosis may occur when there is excessive gastrointestinal or renal bicarbonate loss. Replacement of some of the chloride ions in the feed with acetate or lactate, which are metabolised to bicarbonate, may help to correct the acidosis.

Mild hyponatraemia is common in patients receiving PN and usually does not require an increase in the sodium content of the feed. The cause is often multifactorial and includes increased secretion of vasopressin (antidiuretic hormone) during the stress of acute illness and a decreased ability to maintain accurate fluid balance, particularly in the presence of a high osmolar load being delivered intravenously. Additional sodium and water should be given if there is an obvious source of loss, for example from a fistula or drain. However, if hyponatraemia is secondary to ascites or oedema, the sodium and water content should be decreased. Hypernatraemia can be a manifestation of sodium excess or water deficiency.

DISTURBANCES OF CALCIUM, PHOSPHATE AND MAGNESIUM HOMEOSTASIS

Hypercalcaemia can occur, particularly in patients receiving long-term PN that includes vitamin D and in patients who are immobile. Hypocalcaemia can occur if the content of the feed is inadequate, particularly in the presence of hypomagnesaemia. For physicochemical reasons, the amounts of calcium and magnesium that can be accommodated in a parenteral feed may have to be limited in order to maintain stability. Hypomagnesaemia can also occur secondarily to gastrointestinal loss, e.g. from fistulae, or renal loss, e.g. as a side effect of diuretic therapy. Hypophosphataemia occurs most frequently at the initiation of feeding as a result of rapid cellular uptake.

REFEEDING SYNDROME

The refeeding syndrome comprises the metabolic disturbances that can occur when malnourished patients are aggressively refed. The clinical manifestations of the refeeding syndrome are related to hypophosphataemia, hypokalaemia, hypomagnesaemia, retention of sodium and vitamin deficiencies. The syndrome has been described in association with oral, enteral and parenteral nutrition.

The metabolic abnormalities that occur in the refeeding syndrome have widespread effects including disturbances of cardiovascular, pulmonary, neurological and haematological systems. During prolonged starvation, metabolic pathways are switched from using glucose as a major energy source to using ketones; there is a decrease in basal metabolic rate and insulin secretion. When carbohydrate feeding is reintroduced, glucose again becomes the main source of energy, there is a high demand for phosphate to make intermediates and products of the glycolytic pathway such as fructose 1,6-bisphosphate and ATP, and hypophosphataemia can result. Insulin released in response to the glucose causes potassium and magnesium to move into cells. Magnesium is required for the action of Na^+,K^+-ATPase; hypomagnesaemia, if uncorrected, may cause resistant hypokalaemia. Hyponatraemia may also be part of the refeeding syndrome. It is multifactorial in origin but fluid retention due to an antidiuretic effect of insulin is thought to be important. Thiamin is essential for carbohydrate metabolism as a cofactor for pyruvate dehydrogenase, which converts lactate to pyruvate. Refeeding can increase the demand for thiamin and precipitate deficiency associated with a lactic acidosis.

It is important to anticipate and thus avoid the refeeding syndrome when commencing nutrition support. Patients at particular risk are those with a BMI <16 kg/m^2, unintentional weight loss of more than 15% in the previous 3-6 months, minimal nutritional intake for more than ten days or low plasma potassium, phosphate or magnesium concentrations prior to commencing nutrition support. In such patients, nutrition support should be started slowly using less than the estimated energy requirement, increasing gradually over several days. Generous provision of potassium, phosphate, magnesium and thiamin should be ensured.

LIVER DISEASE
After 2-4 weeks of PN therapy it is common to find increases in plasma bilirubin concentration and liver enzyme activities, particularly transaminases and alkaline phosphatase, which resolve on its discontinuation. Prolonged PN is associated with more marked changes, which include steatosis, fibrosis and cirrhosis. Steatohepatitis may occur as a result of the production of lipid from excess carbohydrate and possibly due to relative choline deficiency. A reduction of total intravenous energy may result in improvement. Cholestasis associated with PN tends to be most severe in those patients who are not receiving any enteral feed to stimulate intestinal motility and maintain secretion of trophic hormones. Improvement may result from treatment with metronidazole to attenuate intestinal flora, ursodeoxycholic acid to modify the consistency of the bile and carnitine to maximise hepatic fatty acid oxidation. Progression to severe and sometimes irreversible liver disease is rare in adults but occurs more frequently in infants and children, possibly owing to physiological cholestasis, less well established antioxidant defences and the different PN formulations used. Long-term PN is associated with both cholelithiasis and acalculous cholecystitis. The risk of these conditions developing may be lessened by stimulating gall bladder contraction with concomitant enteral feeding or cholecystokinin injections.

Hypertriglyceridaemia can occur in patients receiving PN, particularly those with coexisting diabetes mellitus, renal failure, hepatic disease or pancreatitis.

METABOLIC BONE DISEASE

Metabolic bone disease has been described as a complication of long-term PN and may present with bone pain, as radiological evidence of demineralisation or as biochemical abnormalities. Structurally it may appear as deficient calcification or as a decreased bone mass. Its cause is unclear and probably multifactorial, possible aetiological factors including deficiency of some PN components such as vitamins D and K, and toxicity of others, e.g. aluminium. Other factors predisposing to bone disease include those related to the illnesses leading to the requirement for PN and their associated treatments, e.g. low body weight, amenorrhoea or corticosteroids.

Surgical alternatives to parenteral nutrition

In a very few patients, attempts to provide adequate long-term nutrition through PN are unsuccessful. Causes include impending liver failure, limited venous access or frequent episodes of severe dehydration. Such patients with PN failure may be candidates for intestinal surgery. Surgical interventions that have been used in the management of chronic intestinal failure include procedures to restore intestinal continuity, improve residual function and increase the functional length of the intestine.

Transplantation procedures may replace just the gut, both the liver and intestine (as may be required in patients with PN-induced liver damage) or involve multiple visceral transplantation. Indications for the latter procedure include splanchnic vascular thrombosis and extensive gastrointestinal polyposis. Developments in immunosuppressive agents and better graft survival are increasing the range of patients for whom abdominal visceral transplantation is a potential therapeutic option. Survival after transplantation now exceeds 75% at one year and 40% at 10 years, with over 90% of survivors achieving nutritional autonomy.

Conclusion

The incidence of malnutrition is high, particularly in hospital patients, and many require nutrition support. This can be provided as oral supplements or via enteral or parenteral feeding. The need for nutrition support is usually temporary, although in some patients it is lifelong and requires careful monitoring with appropriate laboratory testing.

Further reading

Elia M. Artificial nutrition support. Medicine International 1990; **82:** 3392-3396. *(Note: reference for the Elia nomogram).*

McKee R. Artificial nutrition and nutritional support in hospital. Medicine 2006; **34:** 543-547.

National Institute for Health and Clinical Excellence 2006. Nutrition support in adults (www.nice.org.uk/page.aspx?o=cg032fullguideline).

Rombeau JL, Rolandelli RH (Eds). Clinical Nutrition: Parenteral Nutrition (3rd edition). Philadelphia, USA: Saunders, 2001.

Smith T, Elia M. Artificial nutrition support in hospital: indications and complications. Clinical Medicine 2006; **5:** 457-460.

Chapter 6

Obesity

Introduction

Obesity in adults is defined as a body mass index (BMI) > 30 kg/m^2 (weight divided by the square of the height). This is a useful measurement as it is easily obtained and has been used in most of the studies on which knowledge of the health effects of obesity is based. However, BMI takes no account of the distribution of body fat or of variation with ethnic group, age or gender (see Chapter 4). Waist circumference measurement can also be used as a measure of obesity. It provides a marker of abdominal fat stores that gives an indication of long-term health risks, particularly in relation to cardiovascular disease. In children, the definition of obesity is more difficult and associated morbidities are less well documented. A useful definition of obesity in children is a weight ≥ 95th centile for BMI for age. A further definition of obesity, useful for clinical although not epidemiological purposes, is those patients with weight related comorbidity.

Prevalence

The prevalence of obesity in the UK has increased from 6% of men and 8% of women in 1980 to 23.6 and 23.8% respectively in 2004. Between 1993 and 2002, the percentage of adults either overweight or obese increased from 57.6 to 69.1 for men and from 48.6 to 58.5 for women. Between 1995 and 2003, the percentage of children aged 2-10 years either obese or overweight increased from 22.7% in 1995 to 27.7%. Obesity in boys increased from 9.6% to 14.9% and in girls from 10.3% to 12.5%. If these trends continue it is estimated that over one third of adults and 50% of children will be obese by 2020.

Normal regulation of energy intake and expenditure

Body weight tends to remain relatively constant despite variations in daily energy expenditure and in food intake. A complex mechanism exists to control body weight, which balances energy intake and expenditure through afferent signals and efferent effects (Figure 6.1).

When food is readily available, hunger leads to eating. Satiety signals then result in a feeling of fullness and intake ceases. High energy intake leads to increased energy storage unless energy expenditure is increased. Within the brain, satiety signals are integrated with signals of long-term energy status in order to bring about a response to current nutritional status. This response is effected by food-seeking behaviour, changes in energy expenditure and alterations in metabolic pathways concerned with energy storage.

Multiple factors are involved in the regulation of food intake, some even prior to ingestion. For example, the sight, smell and even memory of food have effects that include increased salivation and gastrointestinal hormone secretion.

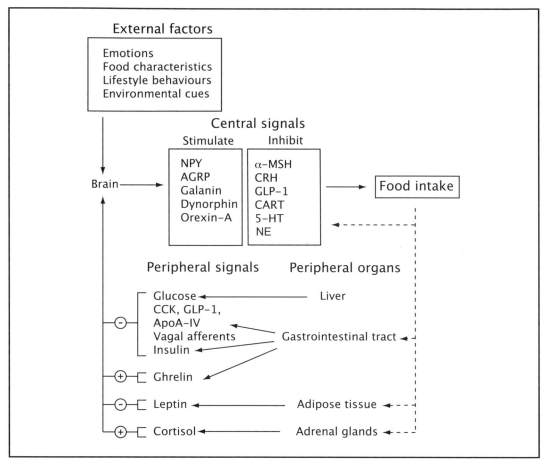

Figure 6.1 Regulation of food intake; see text for expansion of abbreviations

Central regulation of food intake

The brainstem and hypothalamus are integral to the control of energy balance. The arcuate nucleus within the hypothalamus is of particular importance as it receives peripheral signals and integrates them through two opposing systems of peptides. One system (orexigenic) stimulates food intake via neuropeptide Y (NPY) and agouti related protein (AGRP); the other system (anorexigenic) inhibits food intake via pro-opiomelanocortin (POMC) and cocaine and amphetamine-regulated transcript (CART). The maintenance of food intake is essential and more than one system exists to ensure it is able to continue.

OREXIGENIC PEPTIDES

Neuropeptide Y is widely distributed within the nervous system; hypothalamic concentrations reflect nutritional status. In addition to increasing food intake, experimental administration of NPY results in decreased thermogenesis, hyper-cortisolism and insulin resistance. Neuropeptide Y is part of the pancreatic polypeptide family, which includes peptide YY (PYY) and pancreatic polypeptide (PP); these also have effects on energy balance.

Endogenous opioids are also involved in the central control of energy balance. β-endorphin, a product of the POMC gene, is localised in the arcuate nucleus. Other opioids, including leucine-enkephalin and methionine-enkephalin, are widely distributed in the hypothalamus. The effect of opioids on feeding appears to be modest and of short duration but they may have a role in the reward pathways associated with food, together with dopamine and serotonin. There is also evidence suggesting that cannabinoids and their receptors (endocannabinoids) may be involved in these reward pathways.

ANOREXIGENIC SIGNALS

αMelanocyte-stimulating hormone (αMSH) is a product of the POMC gene. It acts as an agonist of the melanocortin receptors MC3-R and MCH-R, which are impor-tant in regulating food intake. Cocaine and amphetamine-regulated transcript (CART) is co-expressed with αMSH in the arcuate nucleus and acts in such a way as to inhibit the NPY stimulated feeding response. Agouti related protein is co-expressed with NPY and is an endogenous antagonist of the melanocortin system; as such it is orexigenic.

Some peptides previously thought to be localised to the gastrointestinal tract have been found to be expressed in the hypothalamus, including glucagon-like peptide 1 and ghrelin; these peptides may act as central anorexigenic signals.

Peripheral regulation

Various factors are involved in the peripheral regulation of energy balance. Meal size is largely determined by satiety brought about by mechanoreceptors and chemoreceptors in the gut, acting through the vagal nerves, and by the action of gut peptides. The peptide ghrelin stimulates eating: other gut peptides tend to have an inhibitory effect (Figure 6.2).

GUT HORMONES

Ghrelin is a peptide containing 28 amino acids that is secreted mainly from the stomach. It is also expressed in the brainstem and hypothalamic nuclei and is the endogenous ligand for the growth hormone secretagogue receptor, although its endocrine and weight-regulatory actions are thought to be distinct. In animal

Hormones involved in peripheral regulation of energy balance

Site of secretion	Hormone
Gut	Ghrelin
	Peptide YY (PYY)
	Glucagon-like peptide 1 (GLP-1)
	Cholecystokinin (CCK)
Adipose tissue	Leptin
	Adiponectin
	Resistin
Pancreas	Insulin
Other tissues	Thyroxine
	Cortisol

Figure 6.2 Hormones involved in peripheral regulation of energy balance

studies, ghrelin stimulates appetite and in chronic administration induces obesity. In humans, plasma ghrelin concentrations are increased during fasting and fall during eating, underlying its role as a stimulus to feeding.

Peptide YY (PYY) is produced mainly in the distal intestine, in proportion to the energy ingested. It inhibits appetite by binding to the NPY receptors in the arcuate nucleus. Glucagon-like peptide 1 (GLP-1) and oxyntomodulin arise from processing of the preproglucagon gene in the gut and brain. GLP-1 is released after eating and acts on the pancreas, releasing insulin. Oxyntomodulin is thought to act via the GLP-1 receptor although the mechanism may be different from that of GLP-1 itself.

Cholecystokinin (CKK) stimulates gut motility, pancreatic secretion and gall bladder contraction. In addition, it inhibits food intake by its action on the brain stem. Pancreatic polypeptide (PP) is produced in the gut and pancreas and is thought to play a role in appetite control, possibly via the brainstem pathways. Hormones released by other tissues, including the pancreas and adipose tissue, are also concerned with energy balance.

INSULIN

Insulin was the first adiposity signal to be described, its plasma concentration being noted to vary with body fat mass. Insulin can cross the blood-brain barrier and then act to decrease energy intake. As the primary role of insulin is control of plasma glucose, its concentration tends to fluctuate post prandially so it is able to indicate both short and longer term energy balance.

LEPTIN

Leptin is a 146 amino acid hormone, the product of the *Lep* (formerly *ob*) gene. It is produced by adipocytes in proportion to body weight and thus acts as an appetite regulation signal. Leptin interacts with the arcuate nucleus by stimulating anorexigenic and inhibiting orexigenic neurones. Food restriction decreases leptin concentration, an effect that is reversed by refeeding; hence its function is thought to be to signal low energy levels in conditions of starvation and high energy levels in conditions of plenty, acting across a rather longer timeframe than the gut hormones.

Animal models have been useful in understanding the pathophysiology of leptin. The *ob/ob* mouse is leptin deficient and is obese with hyperinsulinaemia and hyperphagia. Administration of leptin to such mice normalises the phenotype. The *db/db* mouse has a similar phenotype but has an abnormal leptin receptor; circulating plasma leptin concentrations are high, so leptin administration is an ineffective treatment. While a subset of obese humans has relative leptin deficiency, the majority have high circulating plasma leptin concentrations, suggesting leptin resistance and little potential for treatment.

Resistin is also secreted from adipose tissue and may act on it to decrease insulin resistance, although its role is at present unclear. Adiponectin is a complement-like protein. Although it is secreted from adipose tissue, its plasma concentration is lower in obese than lean individuals. It has a role in glucose and lipid metabolism and may protect against insulin resistance.

Other hormones involved indirectly in weight regulation include glucocorticoids and thyroid hormones. Hyperthyroidism tends to result in weight loss (despite increased appetite) and hypothyroidism in weight gain. Adrenal failure leads to weight loss whereas glucocorticoid excess is characterised by gross truncal obesity. These effects are related to changes in both energy intake and expenditure.

Causes of obesity

Obesity is determined by genetic, environmental and behavioural factors that affect energy expenditure and intake. There are rare types of obesity that are inherited in a Mendelian pattern but obesity is more frequently a polygenic trait.

Increased energy intake

Surveys suggest that significant changes in dietary habits have occurred associated with increased obesity. These include increased energy intake between meals and an increase in the percentage of the diet consumed as fat, which is more energy dense and less satiating than protein and carbohydrate. The documented increase in consumption of restaurant and take-away meals may be responsible for an increase in energy intake at mealtimes.

Decreased energy expenditure
Increasing obesity is associated with decreasing physical activity. Technology has facilitated travel and domestic chores and provided new sedentary leisure pursuits; the percentage of the population engaging in planned exercise is decreasing.

Genetic
Estimates of heritability use twin studies to assess the phenotypic variance that is attributable to genetic variation, and have found that for body fat mass this is 40-70%. If obesity is a polygenic trait in a proportion of patients, over which environmental factors have particular influence, this has important implications for treatment strategies. One possible explanation for an interaction of genes and environment is the 'thrifty genotype hypothesis'. This proposes that man evolved in an environment in which food was scarce and survival mechanisms became programmed towards protecting against lack of food. A 'thrifty genotype' would have been a survival advantage then, but in the modern environment would predispose to obesity.

CHROMOSOMAL DISORDERS
Obesity is part of various syndromic disorders, often in association with dysmorphism, mental retardation and organ-specific abnormalities. Examples include Prader-Willi, Down and Bardet-Biedl syndromes and Albright hereditary osteodystrophy (pseudohypoparathyroidism).

Prader-Willi syndrome
Prader-Willi syndrome (PWS) is the most common syndromic cause of obesity, having an incidence of about 1 in 25 000 live births. It is caused by lack of expression of the paternal segment of a gene on chromosome 15 due to a deletion or uniparental disomy. In the neonatal period, children with PWS usually require artificial feeding, but from about one year of age, hyperphagia and obesity develop. The increase and distribution of body fat mass resembles that of growth hormone deficiency and abnormal growth hormone response to stimulation supports hypothalamic dysfunction as the cause. Growth hormone is an effective treatment for these patients, promoting growth, decreasing total body fat and increasing lean body mass. Hyperphagia in PWS may be the result of elevated ghrelin, possibly related to its role as a growth hormone secretagogue in a

disturbed hypothalamus rather than to gastrointestinal secretion.

Congenital leptin deficiency
This was first described in two cousins in a consanguineous Pakistani family. They were found to have undetectable leptin concentrations and this was later shown to be caused by a homozygous mutation in the *ob* gene. Characteristic features in these and subsequent patients include a normal birth weight, hyperphagia and early onset obesity, and impaired T cell immunity. Treatment with subcutaneous recombinant leptin suppressed food intake and decreased BMI.

Pro-opiomelanocortin deficiency
Children with mutations in the POMC gene have also presented with normal birth weights but early onset obesity. In addition, they may show evidence of adrenal failure and have pale skin and red hair owing to the lack of ACTH and MSH, which are both derived from POMC.

Melanocortin receptor defects
Mutations in the MC4R are the most common monogenic cause of obesity, estimated to occur in 2.5% of patients with a BMI > 30. They are associated with increased BMI, hyperphagia and hyperinsulinism. Heterozygotes appear to have an intermediate form of the disorder.

Infectious agents in obesity
Infection has been postulated to have a role in obesity. A number of pathogens have been implicated in animal models; for example, the canine distemper virus has been shown to increase body weight and fat cell size and number in mice, and a syndrome has been described in chickens associated with Rous-associated virus-7, characterised by stunting, hyperlipidaemia and obesity. Human adenovirus Ad-36 has been shown to promote adiposity in chickens. SMAM-1 avian adenovirus and human adenovirus Ad-6 have been associated with obesity in humans, although a causal relationship has not been established.

Pre-adipocytes are able to function like macrophages, showing phagocytic and microbicidal activity, and hormones such as leptin, secreted from adipocytes, are able to influence the immune response via actions on T cells and cytokine production. It is therefore feasible that pathogens could stimulate immune modulating factors, which could result in the growth of adipocytes.

Complications of obesity

There is a curvilinear relationship between BMI and mortality. Various complications are associated with obesity (Figure 6.3) and their nature and extent can be influenced by the extent and distribution of the adipose tissue. Patients with a predominantly intra-abdominal fat distribution tend to be at particular risk for cardiovascular complications.

Complications of obesity

Type 2 diabetes mellitus

Cardiovascular system
    Hypertension
    Stroke
    Heart failure
    Myocardial infarction
    Angina
    Peripheral vascular disease
    Cardiomyopathy

Respiratory system
    Breathlessness
    Sleep apnoea

Gastrointestinal system
    Reflux
    Hepatic steatosis
    Gallstones
    Haemorrhoids

Obstetric and gynaecological
    Hypertension
    Fetal abnormality
    Gestational diabetes
    Infertility/hyperandrogenism

Malignancies
    Colon
    Breast
    Prostate
    Uterus, ovary
    Kidney

Psychiatric disorder

Degenerative joint disease

Cataracts

Figure 6.3 Complications of obesity

Metabolic syndrome

The metabolic syndrome is a group of inter-related risk factors that predict those individuals at increased risk of cardiovascular disease and type 2 diabetes mellitus. In the USA, the condition affects 40% of people over 60 years old of whom 84% have abdominal obesity; the diagnostic criteria are shown in Figure 6.4. The metabolic syndrome is the result of hyperinsulinaemia, affected individuals being resistant to the effects of insulin, usually without overt diabetes mellitus. Increased insulin is required to overcome insulin resistance in muscle and adipose tissue, and this has detrimental effects on those tissues that retain normal sensitivity to insulin. Insulin resistance inhibits glucose disposal in muscle and alters the lipolytic response within adipocytes. The resulting increase in plasma free fatty acids, together with the increased concentration of insulin, stimulates the secretion of triglycerides by the liver.

Definition of the metabolic syndrome (2005)	
Central obesity	Defined as waist circumference ≥ 94 cm for Europid men, ≥ 80 cm for women, with ethnic specific values for other groups
Plus any two of the following:	
raised triglycerides	≥ 1.7 mmol/L or specific treatment for this lipid abnormality
reduced HDL cholesterol	< 1.03 mmol/L in males, < 1.29 mmol/L in females or specific treatment for this lipid abnormality
raised blood pressure	Systolic BP ≥ 130 or diastolic ≥ 85 mm Hg or treatment of previously diagnosed hypertension
raised fasting plasma glucose	≥ 5.6 mmol/L or previously diagnosed type 2 diabetes mellitus

Figure 6.4 International Diabetes Federation (IDF) definition of the metabolic syndrome (2005)

Insulin resistance is associated with inflammatory changes in blood vessel walls, which is another potential mechanism for cardiovascular damage. This inflammation can be detected as small increases in inflammatory markers such as C-reactive protein (CRP). Other vascular markers, e.g. plasminogen activator inhibitor-1 (PAI-1) and fibrinogen also correlate positively with increasing obesity.

Polycystic ovarian syndrome (PCOS) is associated with the metabolic syndrome and is thought to be the end result of the effect of an increased amount of insulin acting on ovaries that retain normal insulin sensitivity. Increased ovarian androgen secretion, coupled with a decrease in SHBG occurring secondarily to hyperinsulinism, can result in a significant increase in free testosterone, leading to hirsuitism.

Cardiovascular disease

Obesity increases the risk of cardiovascular disease. Mortality from cardiovascular disease is increased by about 50% in the obese and 90% in the morbidly obese. Contributing factors include the increased prevalence of hyperlipidaemia and hypertension. The hyperlipidaemia is usually a mixed type with increased triglyceride, total cholesterol and low-density lipoprotein (LDL) concentrations and reduced high-density lipoprotein (HDL) concentration. The prevalence of hypertension in obese adults is approximately three times that in the non-obese population. The aetiology of obesity-related hypertension is multifactorial; suggested mechanisms include activation of the sympathetic nervous system by insulin, renal sodium retention and direct pressure on the kidneys.

There is a weaker association between obesity and the risk of stroke. It may be that other associations of stroke, such as serious intercurrent illness and hence potentially low BMI, may mask any effect from obesity. In patients with long-standing obesity, fatty infiltration of the myocardium can occur, leading to cardiomyopathy.

Respiratory disorders

A number of patients with obesity complain of breathlessness; in many it is a manifestation of lack of fitness. However, with increasing obesity, fat deposition in the chest wall, abdomen and upper airways can hinder respiration. The result is decreased diaphragmatic movement, ventilation-perfusion imbalance and an increase in the work of breathing, all leading to breathlessness. The most extreme manifestation of this is sleep apnoea, in which breathing is obstructed during sleep, leading to brief apnoeic episodes with hypoxia and frequent awakenings. The consequence of this is excessive sleepiness during the day. Severe sleep apnoea can lead eventually to increased pulmonary artery pressure, pulmonary hypertension and cor pulmonale, known as Pickwickian syndrome. The use of continuous positive airway pressure ventilation (CPAP) during the night may be helpful in preventing and relieving the symptoms of sleep apnoea.

Malignancy

Obesity is associated with an increased risk of certain tumours. However, there is little research examining the effect of weight loss; this is in part due to the complex nature of confounding factors. Endometrial cancer is increased in obese pre- and postmenopausal women and breast cancer in obese postmenopausal women, a possible explanation being decreased SHBG and increased aromatisation of oestrogen that occurs in adipose tissue. Carcinoma of the biliary tree is also increased in obese women. Renal cell cancer is associated with obesity in men and women. Colon cancer has a strong positive association with BMI in men and a weaker association in women, being particularly correlated with abdominal obesity. Dietary components may be involved in these associations, for example a diet low in fruit, vegetables and fibre and high in simple carbohydrates predisposes to colon cancer.

Reproductive disorders

In addition to an association with PCOS, hyperandrogenism is common in obese women, secondary to steroid metabolism in adipose tissue. Hyperinsulinism may increase ovarian androgen production and decrease SHBG. This may lead to hirsuitism, amenorrhoea and infertility. Obese women have an increased risk of obstetric complications, including pregnancy-induced hypertension, gestational diabetes and caesarian section. An increased risk of neural tube defects has been reported in fetuses of women with a BMI $> 29 \text{ kg}/\text{m}^2$.

Fatty liver

Fatty infiltration of the liver (non-alcoholic fatty liver disease or NAFLD) may occur secondarily to inhibition of fatty acid oxidation by insulin, particularly in abdominal obesity. This is often recognised clinically as an increase in trans-aminase activity or by changes on ultrasound examination. The process is usually benign, although it may have an effect on liver function, thus leaving patients more susceptible to the effect of drugs and toxins. A minority develop inflammatory changes (non-alcoholic steatotic hepatitis or NASH), a few of whom progress to cirrhosis and eventually end stage liver disease.

Gall bladder disease

Gallstones are associated with obesity, secondary to hepatic oversecretion of cholesterol into the bile.

Degenerative joint disease

The obese have an increased incidence of degenerative joint disease (osteoarthritis) particularly of weight-bearing joints such as the knee and hip. This is of particular significance in that the associated pain tends to limit the ability to exercise, thus affecting the potential for future weight loss. In addition, joint replacement operations carry increased morbidity and mortality rates in the obese and may be contraindicated for this reason.

Cataracts

There is an association between cataracts and obesity. This may be an independent effect or via an association with diabetes mellitus or hypertension.

Treatment of obesity

Population-based treatment

Major public health campaigns, notably in Finland, have been effective in promoting healthy eating and have been associated with weight loss and delay in the development, or possibly prevention, of diabetes. It may be that an approach targeting groups of patients at high risk would be successful in the UK. Children are often considered suitable for such public health programmes but older adults and the elderly should also be considered.

Individual treatment

The aim of obesity treatment is to improve health by reducing to, and then maintaining, an acceptable body weight. To be successful, this ideally requires a multidisciplinary team approach to help the patient make changes in behaviour, physical activity and diet. Pharmacotherapy and surgery may be required in severe cases.

Prior to treatment, patients should undergo evaluation including clinical history, examination and appropriate laboratory investigation. The extent of the obesity and any associated complications such as hypertension or hyperandrogenism should be noted. Evaluation also enables identification of any contributing factors, e.g. genetic abnormalities (such as Prader-Willi syndrome), endocrine disease (such as Cushing's) or psychiatric disorders, such as binge eating or depression.

In order to determine management, any previous treatment must be elicited and a suitable patient-specific plan agreed. Many patients have already attempted self-directed dieting prior to seeking medical help. The role of the multidisciplinary team is to provide motivation, information and support to bring about successful weight loss. Patients' own weight goals are often unrealistic; a suitable target is to lose 10% of body weight in six months. An energy deficit of about 7000 kcal is required for the loss of 1 kg of fat.

Lifestyle changes and treatment of comorbidities

In addition to weight loss, lifestyle changes and therapy can be introduced to address risk factors known to be associated with obesity-related morbidity and mortality. These risk factors include smoking, hypertension, hyperlipidaemia and dysglycaemia, alone or as part of the metabolic syndrome. The requirement for treatment may decline with weight loss.

While all patients should be urged to stop smoking, this is particularly relevant in the obese owing to the association of smoking with vascular disease and possibly an increased risk of type 2 diabetes.

Many obese patients require treatment for hypertension. Although lifestyle change and dietary salt restriction may be implemented, ACE inhibitors, angiotensin II receptor blockers and calcium channel blockers tend to be the first line treatments. Thiazide diuretics can increase plasma glucose and uric acid, often already high in metabolic syndrome, and β-blockers may also increase the risk of diabetes.

If dyslipidaemia is present, statins are usually the drug of choice, some trials having shown that, in addition to improving the lipid profile, they decrease vascular events and the onset of type 2 diabetes, and may improve renal function and reduce plasma uric acid concentrations.

Type 2 diabetes should be treated by conventional means. No drugs are licensed to treat insulin resistance with euglycaemia, but metformin, meglitinides (e.g. nateglinide and repaglinide) and thiazolidinediones (e.g. pioglitazone and rosiglitazone), show promise in reducing progression to type 2 diabetes mellitus.

Exercise
Exercise is prescribed as part of weight loss regimens to redress the imbalance between energy intake and expenditure, yet the recommendations tend not to be evidence-based. Exercise can enhance the treatment of obesity by decreasing appetite and by increasing energy expenditure. Very strenuous exercise temporarily depresses appetite, possibly owing to diversion of gastrointestinal blood flow to muscle, and there may be beneficial effects from lesser degrees of exercise on appetite, e.g. appetite suppression by catecholamines.

Exercise-induced increase in energy expenditure can occur during exercise or can persist after it has finished. Assuming a requirement of 100 kcal to walk one mile, 70 miles must be walked to lose 1 kg. However, in those who are fit, exercise can increase the resting energy expenditure for up to 24 h. An increase of 10% in resting energy expenditure in a 100 kg patient could amount to 240 kcal/24 h. Aerobic, but not resistance, exercise has been shown to produce only modest weight loss but is of additional benefit in combination with diet. In addition, in patients who combine exercise with dieting, more fat and less lean tissue is lost.

The role of exercise is particularly important for successful weight maintenance, although the exact prescription is undecided. 2000 kcal per week of physical activity has been suggested for maintenance of weight loss, which equates to approximately seven hours of brisk walking; others suggest ten hours per week.

The type of exercise may also be important, with bursts of high intensity exercise being expected to have the most effect on appetite and resting energy expenditure and longer periods of lower intensity exercise having a greater effect on fat oxidation. In practice, the nature of any exercise undertaken is probably best dictated by the patient to ensure compliance.

Behavioural modification

Behavioural modification can be useful as part of a weight loss programme helping patients to achieve and maintain weight loss. Techniques include showing patients how to monitor environmental cues that trigger eating, stress management and maximising social support.

Dietary therapy

FASTING

Fasting is not recommended for weight reduction. It leads to excessive loss of lean tissue and to ketone formation. In addition, compensatory changes occur resulting in decreased energy expenditure and physical effort, thus reducing its anticipated benefit.

VERY LOW CALORIE DIETS

Very low calorie diets (VLCD) with an energy content of < 800 kcal/24 h are usually reserved for the morbidly obese when conventional diets have failed. Such diets have a relatively high protein content to maintain lean body mass, (usually at least 28% of energy content), with a low carbohydrate and very low fat content. A 12 week VLCD regimen is often followed by a gradual transition to a balanced diet. As well as allowing behavioural adjustment, this reduces weight change due to shifts in water balance secondary to restoration of glycogen stores. While VLCDs produce greater initial weight loss than low calorie diets (LCDs), their advantage in the long term is unclear.

LOW CALORIE DIETS

Low calorie diets of 1000-1200 kcal/24 h for women and 1200-1600 kcal/24 h for men result in average weight loss of 0.5-1.0 kg per week. Personalised eating plans can be drawn up by a dietitian mindful of a patient's food preferences, budget and social circumstances. Commercial weight loss programmes such as Weight Watchers, run by a successful 'graduate', are widely available and some incorporate the use of proprietary meal replacements as liquids, bars and ready meals.

LOW GLYCAEMIC INDEX DIETS

The glycaemic index (GI) refers to the blood glucose response to the ingestion of a food compared with the ingestion of a reference food. Low GI foods, such as wholegrain cereals and fruit, are absorbed slowly, which may reduce insulin release and the metabolic response, leading to increased satiety and hence a decreased energy intake.

HIGH PROTEIN DIETS

High protein diets, for example the Atkins diet, are similar to low GI regimens in that they are intended to suppress insulin secretion. They contain about 25% of energy as protein, 70% as fat and as little as 5% as carbohydrate. High protein diets induce ketosis, which may contribute to loss of appetite and hence their relative popularity despite little objective evidence of their superiority over other dieting strategies. There are some concerns over the use of high protein diets. In particular, they tend to have high contents of saturated fat and sodium, which increase cardiovascular risk, and dietary intake of purines may also be high, which increases plasma urate concentration, a predisposing factor for gout.

Pharmacotherapy

Pharmacotherapy has tended to be reserved for the short-term treatment of resistant obesity in patients with a BMI $\geq$ 30, or for patients with a BMI of 27-29 in the presence of at least one major comorbidity. However, the rapid increase in the prevalence of obesity and the chronicity of the condition may lead to widening of these indications. There are few contraindications to the use of drugs in the treatment of obesity, although they should be avoided in pregnancy and lactation, in systemic illness and unstable psychiatric disorders. A history of anorexia nervosa is an absolute contraindication. Possible mechanisms of action of anti-obesity drugs are shown in Figure 6.5.

Mechanisms of action of anti-obesity agents	
Reduction of energy intake	Decreased hunger/appetite
	Increased satiety
	Altered fat and/or carbohydrate preference
	Decreased nutrient absorption
Increase in energy expenditure	Stimulation of physical activity
	Increased metabolic rate

Figure 6.5 Mechanisms of action of anti-obesity agents

REDUCTION OF ENERGY INTAKE

Amphetamine is a β-phenethylamine that interferes with dopaminergic neuro-transmission. It was developed as a stimulant drug to treat narcolepsy. Its ability to produce weight loss was realised, but its stimulant properties (and the potential for addiction) made prescription for this purpose unsuitable and led to the production of derivatives for use as anti-obesity agents. Phentermine, diethylpropion and mazindol were phenethylamines developed for the treatment of obesity and while they had lower abuse potential than amphetamine, they still had troublesome stimulant side effects and were later withdrawn.

Fenfluramine and dexfenfluramine were then introduced. They were serotonin-ergic agonists effective as anti-obesity agents, which were also associated with a reduction in insulin resistance, improved glucose tolerance and a reduction in blood pressure, independent of weight loss. Fenfluramine may have had an effect in decreasing carbohydrate craving whereas there is some evidence that dexfen-fluramine caused a selective decrease in dietary fat intake. They were withdrawn owing to a link with cardiac valve lesions and pulmonary hypertension.

Sibutramine selectively inhibits the reuptake of noradrenaline, serotonin and, to a lesser extent, dopamine. It produces a reduction in food intake via an effect on satiety and may alter food preferences, tending to decrease fat intake. Sibutramine has a slight thermogenic effect, which may counteract the decrease in metabolic rate that occurs with dieting. The noradrenergic effects can cause hypertension or increased heart rate and in some patients this may be a contraindication to commencing, or a reason to discontinue, treatment.

Orlistat binds to gastric and pancreatic lipases, decreasing the hydrolysis of ingested triglyceride. This results in a dose-dependent partial fat malabsorption. Adverse effects tend to be secondary to fat malabsorption and include abdominal pain, loose stools, faecal urgency and oily discharge. In some patients, the occurrence of such symptoms after eating high fat meals may help the adoption of a lower fat, and usually lower energy, diet.

Acarbose is an inhibitor of pancreatic amylase and brush border α-glucosidase. It decreases absorption of carbohydrate and is used in the treatment of diabetes mellitus. While it might, theoretically, be of use as an anti-obesity agent, it has not been so to date. Other amylase inhibitors from vegetable sources may prove useful in this respect after further development.

INCREASE IN ENERGY EXPENDITURE

Drugs able to increase the metabolic rate and dissipate excess energy as heat, with minimal effect on cardiovascular status, would be ideal as anti-obesity agents.

Thyroid hormones increase metabolic rate and, in excess, cause weight loss. However, they are not therapeutic options as they can cause cardiovascular side effects and tend to be associated with loss of fat free mass. Thyroid hormone analogues, which increased metabolic rate in skeletal muscle but spared cardiac muscle, would potentially make good anti-obesity agents.

Ephedrine increases noradrenergic stimulation and its effect is potentiated by caffeine. The mechanism of weight loss is multifactorial, including increased protein synthesis and brown fat stimulation as a result of β-stimulation, and increased α-receptor mediated conversion of thyroxine to triiodothyronine. Cardiovascular side effects and anxiety are associated with its use.

β_3-Adrenoreceptors mediate the thermogenic effects of sympathomimetics but not the effects on heart rate and smooth muscle. Various synthetic β_3-agonists are being developed for the pharmacotherapy of obesity.

Some medications noted to cause weight loss as a side effect have been investigated in trials but they are not in common use as anti-obesity agents. Cimetidine is a H_2-receptor antagonist developed for the treatment of peptic ulcers, and is thought to have an effect on satiety. Topiramate is an anti-epilepsy agent. It is a carbonic anhydrase inhibitor although the mechanism by which it induces weight loss is unclear. The sulphonamide-type anti-epilepsy drug zonisamide is also effective in causing weight loss. Other medications that have been observed to cause weight loss include bupropion, an antidepressant with adrenergic activity, and bromocriptine, a dopamine agonist used in the treatment of Parkinson's disease.

A number of over-the-counter preparations are sold as slimming aids and in many cases there is no objective evidence of their efficacy. Examples include chitosan, a polysaccharide from the exoskeleton of crustaceans; chromium picolinate, a cofactor for insulin; ma-huang (*Ephedra sinica*), an evergreen shrub, and guar gum, a dietary fibre from the Indian cluster bean. Of these preparations, ma-huang, whose active component is ephedrine, has been associated with weight loss, but is not recommended owing to its adverse effects.

Based on current knowledge of weight-regulating pathways, new approaches to therapy are being developed. Rimonabant (Acomplia) is a selective endocannabinoid receptor blocker, which has been shown to be effective in the treatment of obesity. It suppresses appetite and shows promise in decreasing dependence and habituation associated with food consumption. In theory, leptin would be a potential treatment, yet its efficacy is limited in most obese patients due to leptin resistance or the inability of leptin to cross the blood-brain barrier. Potential pharmacological solutions might include drugs able to sensitise the leptin pathway. As mutations of the MC4 receptor have been found to be a common cause of obesity, receptor antagonists could prove to be a useful therapeutic option. Studies in patients with type 2 diabetes have shown that GLP-1 acts to decrease blood glucose. However, its short half life has restricted clinical use. Exendin is a peptide with 50% homology to GLP-1, obtained from lizard salivary secretions, which, in humans, promotes satiety and weight loss and enhances insulin sensitivity. Theoretically, it may have a role in obese patients with type 2 diabetes.

Bariatric surgery

The use of diet, exercise and drugs as treatments for obesity has not resulted in a marked decrease in its prevalence. However, patients who have surgery as treatment for their obesity (bariatric surgery) are able to achieve and maintain considerable weight loss.

Early bariatric techniques included jaw wiring and jejunoileal bypass. In most patients, jaw wiring resulted in weight loss due to the dietary restrictions imposed by the temporary physical barrier to eating. However, no long lasting reprogramming effects resulted from the enforced lack of chewing and weight tended to be regained quickly following removal of the wires. Jejunoileal bypass involved surgical connection of the proximal jejunum to the distal ileum, bypassing about 90% of the small intestine. Weight loss resulted secondarily to malabsorption but at the price of significant complications, such as severe diarrhoea, electrolyte disturbances, oxalate renal stones and vitamin deficiencies.

Developments in surgical techniques have led to operations being a viable treatment option for many patients. Bariatric surgery is currently recommended in carefully selected patients with a BMI ≥ 40 or between 35 and 40 with significant other disease that might be improved by weight loss, e.g. diabetes or hypertension.

Current surgical procedures for the treatment of obesity are of two types (Figure 6.6): restrictive surgery (i.e. vertical banded gastroplasty or adjustable gastric banding) or malabsorptive surgery (i.e. Roux-en-Y gastric bypass or biliopancreatic diversions).

GASTRIC RESTRICTION

Restrictive procedures were devised to decrease the capacity of the stomach after observations that patients who required subtotal gastrectomy for other indications lost weight. There are two basic techniques for gastric restriction. Vertical banded gastroplasty (VBG) uses staples to create a vertical pouch on the lesser curve of the stomach, the outlet of which is restricted by a band. Adjustable gastric banding (AGB) involves the placing of a silicone band distal to the gastro-oesophageal junction, the inflation of which can be adjusted using a subcutaneous access port.

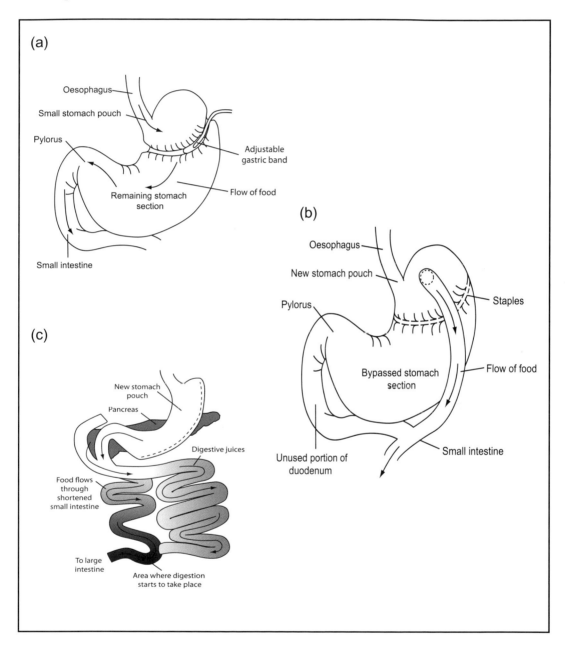

Figure 6.6 Operative procedures of (a) gastric banding, (b) Roux-en-Y gastric bypass and (c) biliopancreatic diversion

MALABSORPTIVE PROCEDURES

The theoretical advantage of malabsorptive procedures is that they allow patients to eat normal sized meals yet weight loss still occurs.

Gastric bypass consists of transection of the stomach coupled with a Roux-en-Y gastrojejunostomy. The stomach contents then bypass the distal stomach and proximal small intestine; the resulting malabsorption contributes to the greater weight loss.

In biliopancreatic diversions, the stomach volume is reduced to 200-500 mL and the remainder anastomosed to the distal small intestine. The excluded small intestine, including the outlets for biliary and pancreatic secretions, is introduced 50 cms proximal to the terminal ileum.

While gastric restriction has mechanical effects and biliopancreatic diversions lead to malabsorption, some of the effectiveness of these procedures is due to perturbations in gut hormones. Peptide YY is increased after gastrojejunal bypass with a potentially anorexic effect. Plasma concentrations of the orexigenic hormone ghrelin fall after gastric bypass procedures, contributing to their effectiveness.

BENEFITS

Bariatric surgery is effective in bringing about weight loss and reducing the complications associated with obesity. Weight loss is maximal between one and a half and two years post-operatively but has been shown to be maintained in the long term. After gastric bypass surgery, the average excess weight loss has been shown to be 75% at five years and more than 50% after ten years.

COMPLICATIONS

The incidence of complications varies according to the nature of the procedure and the centre in which it is being performed. Mortality has been estimated to be 0.14% for restrictive and 0.3-2.5% for malabsorptive operations in the best centres.

Longer term complications may occur and it is necessary for all patients who have had bariatric surgery to be followed up by a multidisciplinary team including a physician, dietitian, surgeon and psychologist.

Nutritional deficiencies

All bariatric surgical operations have a potential risk of nutritional deficiencies due to either malabsorption or to the adoption of altered eating habits. Roux-en-Y gastric bypass increases the risk of iron, vitamin B_{12} and calcium deficiencies. Biliopancreatic diversion can lead to protein energy malnutrition and decreased absorption of fat soluble vitamins and calcium.

Bone disease

Measurement of bone mineral density is difficult in obese patients due to practical issues and lack of validated reference data. However, it is probably greater than average in the majority of obese patients. Rapid loss of weight seems to be associated with a reduction in bone mineral density, although the clinical relevance of this with regard to bariatric surgery is unclear. It is important, particularly in those who have undergone malabsorptive procedures, to ensure adequate vitamin D intake and so prevent calcium malabsorption and reduce the risk of osteoporosis.

Gallstones

Any rapid decrease in weight is associated with increased formation of gallstones. This complication occurs in about 30% of patients who have undergone gastric bypass. Management strategies include removal of the gall bladder at the time of bariatric surgery or prophylactic use of ursodeoxycholic acid.

Excess skin

Substantial weight loss after surgery may leave excess skin folds. Patients find these unsightly and usually request 'cosmetic' surgery at least on the redundant abdominal skin, known as an apron. Rarely, skin folds may be large enough to interfere with mobility or may become ulcerated or infected.

Dumping syndrome

Patients who have had gastric bypass may suffer from symptoms associated with dumping syndrome on eating foods with a high sugar content. This is the result of food with a high osmotic load passing into the small bowel unchecked by the pylorus, which causes abdominal pain. In addition, the resulting insulin release may cause symptomatic hypoglycaemia. For most patients, this complication resolves with time as a result of intestinal adaptation.

Conclusion

Obesity is rapidly increasing in prevalence, owing to changes in lifestyle and genetic predisposition. Increasing knowledge of the complex mechanisms involved in control of energy balance is leading to greater understanding of the underlying genetic abnormalities and providing new prospects for treatment.

Further reading

Arterburn DE, DeLaet DE, Schaeur D. Clinical Evidence: Obesity. www.clinicalevidence.com

Bloom S, Wynne K, Chaudhri O. Gut feeling – the secret of satiety? Clin Med 2005; **5:** 147-152.

Finer N. Obesity. Clin Med 2003; **1:** 23-27.

Wynne K, McGowan B, Bloom S. Appetite control. J Endocrinol 2005; **184**: 291-318.

Chapter 7

Disease-specific nutrition

Introduction

Nutritional intervention is not only of value in diseases related to deficiency or excess of nutrients. There are numerous conditions in which dietary interventions have been proven to have a beneficial role, either alone or in conjunction with other forms of treatment. We review some of the more important of these in this chapter, and also discuss the use of functional foods (foods considered to have benefit beyond those specifically related to their nutrient contents) and nutraceuticals (substances that may be components of a normal diet but of which dietary supplementation may be of value even in the absence of evidence of deficiency).

However, in formulating specific dietary interventions in these conditions, the principles of good nutrition must not be neglected. Interventions must be planned in the context of the overall provision of amounts of nutrients to maintain normal structure and function, in a palatable and digestible form. An intervention that is potentially beneficial in relation to a specific disease may have adverse effects overall.

Cardiovascular disease

Many dietary manipulations may be of value in patients with cardiovascular disease. The role of salt and the possible benefits of dietary salt reduction in hypertension are discussed in Chapter 1 (p.13). Moderate salt restriction is also of potential benefit in patients with cardiac failure (particularly in patients resistant to diuretics), but severe restriction is not required. Alcohol has a negative inotropic effect and alcohol intake should be limited in cardiac failure (although a modest alcohol intake – particularly if taken as red wine – appears to have a beneficial effect on plasma lipid profiles and the risk of coronary artery disease).

Dietary intervention is particularly important in patients with atherosclerosis although it should be emphasised that this is a multifactorial disorder and the approach to its management, whether in relation to primary or secondary prevention, should include attempting to modify all the identifiable risk factors that are susceptible to intervention. However, dietary intervention is of proven value independently of the management of other risk factors.

The principles include normalisation and maintenance of body weight (patients with central obesity are at particularly high risk of cardiovascular disease), reduction of fat intake (particularly saturated and *trans*-unsaturated fats) and cholesterol with a relative increase in the intake of complex carbohydrates and an intake of about 400 g (equivalent to five portions) of fruit and vegetables a day. These are essentially the recommended guidelines for a healthy diet for the great majority of people. The specific recommendations regarding the intake of different forms of fat (within the overall recommendation that it should provide no more than 30% of the total energy intake) are given in Chapter 2 (p.27). Although diets that have a low content of antioxidants are associated with an increased risk of cardiovascular disease, there is no consistent evidence from randomised controlled trials for any benefit from dietary supplementation with antioxidants.

One risk factor for atherosclerosis that has received particular attention with regard to the possibility of dietary intervention is homocysteine. There is persuasive evidence that hyperhomocysteinaemia is an independent risk factor, particularly for coronary disease. Folic acid has an essential role in the metabolism of homocysteine but there is little evidence that increasing the folate content of the diet is beneficial in individuals with high plasma homocysteine concentrations.

Critical illness

Critical illness can provide challenges to the provision of adequate nutrition. Patients are rarely able to eat normally and enteral feeding using a tube may be compromised by immotility of the gut secondary, for example, to the use of muscle relaxant drugs required for the patient to be ventilated, or to electrolyte disturbance. If this is the case, parenteral nutrition will be required, but in the authors' experience only a minority of patients on intensive therapy units require parenteral nutrition.

Estimation of energy requirements is often difficult, particularly if patients are paralysed and ventilated (reducing requirements). Any impairment of renal function may affect the requirement for minerals, particularly, and the use of renal replacement therapy can lead to the loss of vitamins and amino acids from the bloodstream. Dialysis fluids contain glucose and their use may contribute to hyperglycaemia.

Most important, however, are the body's pathophysiological responses to severe illness (sometimes called 'the metabolic response to trauma/stress'). This is a hypercatabolic state leading to negative nitrogen balance with insulin resistance that may lead to hyperglycaemia. There is often fluid retention, and increased capillary permeability will contribute to the fall in plasma albumin concentration that is frequently observed. The provision of nutrition support alone cannot reverse this state. Many therapies, including the use of growth hormone, anabolic steroids and other agents, have been tried but with limited success. The use of growth hormone has been shown to be positively harmful in some studies. The mainstays of treatment are support of vital functions, maintenance of electrolyte and fluid balance and the use of insulin to prevent hyperglycaemia (and possibly for its anabolic effect). Of specific therapies, the use of recombinant human protein C has been shown to be beneficial in some patients.

Although it has been suggested that the use of fat emulsions as an energy source in parenteral nutrition may have adverse effects on pulmonary, renal and immune function in critically ill patients, the evidence is inconsistent and a limited ability to utilise glucose as an energy source mandates the judicious use of fat as well as glucose as an energy source in most patients. Measurement of plasma triglyceride concentrations will indicate whether the fat is being cleared adequately. Supplementation with specific nutrients, e.g. glutamine, arginine, omega-3 unsaturated fatty acids and nucleotides, has been advocated at various times, but has not been proven to be of value in the majority of patients with critical illness. There is, however, promising although not conclusive evidence of the value of glutamine supplementation in patients with burns and severe trauma.

Diabetes mellitus

Dietary management is central to the overall management of diabetes mellitus, both types 1 and 2. The general principles are straightforward: a diet that allows the attainment and maintenance of a body mass index in the healthy range, and which is appropriate for reducing the risk of cardiovascular disease, for which diabetes is a major risk factor. Specific groups of patients will require additional modifications, for example, children and pregnant women, and those with established nephropathy or conditions that interfere with normal gut function, such as cystic fibrosis.

Before the introduction of insulin, the mainstay of the treatment of diabetes was restriction of carbohydrate intake and restriction continued to be recommended for many years afterwards. Given that the protein content of the diet is largely determined by financial considerations rather than availability (at least in developed countries), avoidance of weight loss inevitably meant that the diets recommended for patients with diabetes tended to be high in fat. With the increasing appreciation of both a high dietary fat intake and diabetes as risk factors for cardiovascular disease, dietary recommendations have changed considerably. They are now that the total fat intake should provide not more than 35% of energy requirements, with the bulk of the carbohydrate content being complex carbohydrates (e.g. starches rather than mono- and disaccharides). Similar recommendations are appropriate for patients with impaired glucose tolerance.

Total energy intake

The first step in determining a patient's dietary requirements is to calculate their energy requirements. It is difficult to do this precisely, but it is clearly important to the maintenance of body weight. Patients with newly diagnosed type 1 diabetes may require a higher than calculated intake for a short period if they have experienced significant weight loss. However, many patients with type 2 diabetes are obese, and will require restriction of their energy intake. Furthermore, improvement in glycaemic control may, by reducing glycosuria, contribute to the equation by making more glucose available for storage. Effective patient education is vital: patients all too frequently fail to appreciate that their basal energy requirements will fall as they lose weight. In popular parlance, 'diet' is often regarded as a short term modification of food intake. Diabetes is a lifelong condition: adherence to dietary guidance also needs to be lifelong. Thus patients must be educated to help them achieve a sustained modification of their food intake.

Carbohydrate

That the bulk of dietary carbohydrates should be complex rather than simple carbohydrates has been emphasised above. This reduces the amplitude of the changes in blood glucose concentration that occur between the fasting state and following meals. However, while continuing to be important for patients with type 2 diabetes, it is arguably somewhat less so in type 1 diabetes thanks to modern insulin regimens of the 'basal-bolus' type, where insulin doses are based on the results of frequent blood glucose testing and the anticipated glycaemic response to a particular meal ('carbohydrate counting'). This is the basis of the DAFNE (dose [of insulin] adjustment for normal eating) regimen. Soluble fibre has beneficial effects on glycaemia and lipid metabolism and should be encouraged.

Fat

Although it is recommended that dietary fat intake should provide only 35% of overall energy, in practice, this is often very difficult to achieve and a figure of 35-40% may be more realistic. Saturated and *trans*-unsaturated fats (see p.27) should together provide no more than 10% of total energy intake, as should omega-6 polyunsaturated fat; *cis*-monounsaturated fat should provide 10-20%; an adequate intake of omega-3 polyunsaturated fats should be encouraged through eating oily fish twice a week.

Protein

The recommended protein intake is 50-60 g/day for adult males and 40-50 g/day for females. Some degree of protein restriction may be beneficial in patients with incipient diabetic nephropathy (manifest as microalbuminuria) and a greater degree of protein restriction may be required in established nephropathy.

Special considerations
The dietary recommendations for patients with diabetes must take into account their physiological status, providing, for example, for the increased requirements of growth in children, for the demands of the fetus in pregnancy and lactation during breastfeeding, and for the energy requirements of exercise.

Inherited metabolic diseases
Dietary manipulation is an essential aspect of the management of several inherited metabolic diseases. Many of these manipulations are specific to the disorder, but some diseases, notably cystic fibrosis, put the patient at risk of generalised malnutrition, so that attention to the overall quantity and quality of the nutrient content of the diet is required. It should be appreciated that specific interventions, while designed to be beneficial, may have potentially adverse effects. If accumulation of a substance is responsible for the clinical manifestation of an inherited metabolic disorder, it is logical, and potentially beneficial, to restrict its intake. However, if it is an essential nutrient, its exclusion from the diet will be potentially harmful. An example is the restriction of dietary phenylalanine (an essential amino acid) in phenylketonuria, discussed below.

Dietary strategies in the management of inherited metabolic diseases may involve either restriction of the intake of a nutrient, dietary supplementation, or a combination of both.

Restriction of intake
This is a particularly useful strategy in inherited metabolic diseases in which clinical features are a result of the accumulation of toxic substances. Restriction of dietary phenylalanine in phenylketonuria is the classic example. Were this to be attempted only by restricting overall protein intake, the severity of the restriction required to maintain plasma phenylalanine concentrations within acceptable limits would result in overall protein deficiency. Treatment is thus based on adequate restriction of normal protein intake, coupled with the use of low phenylalanine foods and specific amino acid supplementation. While the principal objective of treatment is to prevent plasma phenylalanine concentrations exceeding toxic concentrations, it is an essential amino acid, so total restriction is not appropriate.

Dihydropteridine reductase deficiency also causes hyperphenylalaninaemia, since the enzyme is required for the recycling of biopterin, a cofactor for phenylalanine hydroxylase, the deficient enzyme. Biopterin is also a cofactor for tyrosine and tryptophan hydroxylases, required for the synthesis of L-dopa and

5-hydroxytryptophan, respectively. These are precursors of the neurotransmitters dopamine and serotonin. Dietary management of this condition comprises restriction of phenylalanine and supplementation with dopa and 5-hydroxytryptophan.

Galactosaemia and hereditary fructose intolerance are managed by dietary restriction of galactose and fructose, respectively, but although this imposes a limitation on the range of foods that can be consumed, it does not put the patients at risk of any specific deficiencies as neither sugar is essential to the diet.

A more general example of dietary restriction is demonstrated by the urea cycle disorders. The harmful consequences of these conditions stem from the accumulation of ammonia. The conditions are managed acutely by stopping dietary protein intake. A similar strategy is used in the management of organic acid acidaemias, but in both cases, some dietary protein must be reintroduced within 48-72 h in order to prevent catabolism.

Augmentation of intake

This can take several forms. Glycogen storage disease type 1 (deficiency of glucose 6-phosphatase) puts the affected individual at risk of fasting hypoglycaemia. It is managed by ensuring an adequate dietary content of complex carbohydrates that are broken down only slowly in the gut, together, if necessary, with the provision of enteral carbohydrate feeding (particularly overnight).

Some inherited metabolic disorders are the result of deficiency of an enzyme that has a vitamin (or vitamin-derived) cofactor. Provided that there is some residual activity, dietary supplementation with the vitamin may have a beneficial effect by increasing the flux through the pathway by a mass action effect. The classic example is homocystinuria (deficiency of cystathionine β-synthase). The enzyme requires pyridoxal phosphate as a coenzyme, and some patients with this condition respond to dietary supplementation with pyridoxine. Figure 7.1 presents a summary of inherited metabolic diseases that can be treated by vitamin supplementation.

Liver disease

In patients with either acute or chronic liver failure, reduction of dietary protein intake can reduce the risk of encephalopathy or have a beneficial effect on its development. However, it is important that the restriction is not so severe as to induce catabolism. Patients with chronic liver disease often have poor appetites and attempts further to restrict protein intake may be positively harmful. The mainstay of treatment is evacuation and sterilisation of the large intestine to reduce the formation and uptake of ammonia.

Vitamins that may be of benefit in the management of inherited metabolic diseases

Cofactor	Disorder
Ascorbic acid	Congenital lactic acidosis Glutathione synthetase deficiency Transient tyrosinaemia of the newborn Tyrosinaemia type III
Biotin	Biotinidase deficiency Multiple carboxylase deficiency Propionic acidaemia Pyruvate carboxylase deficiency
Folate	Dihydropteridine reductase deficiency Methionine synthase deficiency Methylene tetrahydrofolate reductase deficiency Uridine monophosphate synthase deficiency
Hydroxycobalamin	Cobalamin disorders Methylmalonic aciduria
Pyridoxine	Homocystinuria (cystathionine β-synthase deficiency) Ornithine aminotransferase deficiency Pyridoxine responsive seizures
Riboflavin	Congenital lactic acidosis Glutaric aciduria type I Multiple acyl-CoA dehydrogenase deficiency
Thiamin	Congenital lactic acidosis Maple syrup urine disease Pyruvate dehydrogenase deficiency
Tocopherol	Glutathione synthetase deficiency
Ubiquinone	Mitochondrial disorders

Figure 7.1 Vitamins that may be of benefit in the management of inherited metabolic diseases

Patients with encephalopathy tend to have low plasma concentrations of branched chain amino acids, and there has been considerable interest in supplementation with these amino acids, either enterally or parenterally according to the route being used for nutrition. However, analysis of all the trial data does not suggest that this is of benefit.

Dietary sodium restriction is of benefit in patients with cirrhosis, both to reduce the risk of the development of ascites and as an adjunct to its management. Low salt diets are often considered bland and hence unappetising, and in practice it may be difficult to achieve significant reduction of intake without compromising overall nutritional status.

Renal disease

Patients with acute renal failure frequently require nutrition support. During the oliguric phase, the most important modifications of nutrient intake are to minimise potassium and restrict sodium intakes. A low protein intake (such as 0.5-0.6 g/kg/24 h) has sometimes been advocated if it is hoped to manage patients conservatively, but it is important to avoid a negative nitrogen balance. In patients receiving renal replacement therapy, it is not usually necessary to restrict nitrogen intake and patients should be given the equivalent of approximately 1 g/kg/24 h protein. In an adequately hydrated patient, an increase in the plasma concentration of urea that is not accompanied by an increase in creatinine suggests excessive provision of nitrogen. An adequate intake of energy as carbohydrate and fat is important to limit catabolism. Vitamin supplements are usually provided.

Dietary protein restriction used to be considered an important aspect of the management of chronic renal failure, but risks causing negative nitrogen balance and current recommendations are to provide a normal amount of protein (0.8-1.0 g/kg/24 h). As in acute renal failure, provision of sufficient energy is essential to prevent excessive catabolism. Dietary restriction of potassium is important and a low sodium intake is usually appropriate except in patients with high sodium losses. Restriction of phosphate intake may appear appropriate, but is difficult to achieve, and oral phosphate binders are usually prescribed. The design of the diet must take into account the patient's own food preferences, and reflect the fact that modification will be required long-term, unless the patient undergoes a successful transplant. The provision of adequate and appropriate nutrition may be hampered by the anorexia that is often part of the uraemic syndrome.

Anaemia is a frequent complication of chronic renal failure. Although often due in large part to reduced production of erythropoietin (and treated successfully with recombinant erythropoietin or darbepoietin, a hyperglycosylated analogue of erythropoietin), it is important to eliminate other causes, e.g. iron deficiency, and to ensure adequate provision of haematinics to support erythropoiesis. It must also be remembered that chronic renal failure is an important risk factor for cardiovascular disease and the fat composition of the diet should reflect this.

Short bowel syndrome

A patient is said to have a short bowel when there is insufficient length of functioning gut for adequate absorption of nutrients and/or fluid and electrolytes such that supplementation is required to prevent the development of undernutrition. Short bowel syndrome (SBS) is likely to occur when less than 200 cm of small intestine is functional.

Types and causes

The most common causes of short bowel syndrome in adults are Crohn's disease, superior mesenteric artery thrombosis and damage secondary to radiation. It is more common in women, perhaps because their intestines tend to be shorter. In children, the most common causes are necrotising enterocolitis and congenital bowel abnormalities.

Whatever the aetiology, the majority of patients with SBS can be divided into two broad groups: those with short bowel and a high output stoma and those with short bowel and a jejunocolic anastomosis. Patients with a jejunostomy and more than 100 cm of residual jejunum tend to be net absorbers of fluid, being able to absorb adequate water and sodium from oral intake. Patients with <100 cm tend to be net secretors, losing more water and sodium from the stoma than is taken orally, the output increasing during the daytime in response to oral intake.

Tolerance to intestinal resection and the potential for adaptation are influenced by the length and nature of the remaining gut. For example, hormones such as cholecystokinin and gastrin, which decrease gastric secretions, are produced in the jejunum and have a feedback effect, thereby reducing gastric secretions. The terminal ileum is responsible for absorption of vitamin B_{12} and bile salts, the latter having a stimulant effect if they pass through to the colon. The ileum also secretes glucagon-like peptides 1 and 2 and neurotensin, which exert trophic actions that are important for ileal adaptation.

The presence of the ileo-caecal valve is advantageous as it slows the flow of small bowel contents into the colon, potentially increasing absorption: it also decreases the risk of entry of colonic bacteria into the remaining small intestine with subsequent bacterial overgrowth. If the colon is preserved it is able to increase its absorptive capacity to as much as 6 L of fluid and 500 kcal/24 h.

Clinical management

NUTRITION

The length of residual bowel enables the degree of resulting malnutrition to be predicted. Parenteral nutrition is required if a patient absorbs less than about one third of oral intake. Typically, for patients with a jejunostomy, net secretors with <200 cm residual bowel require supplemental fluid and those with <150 cm require supplementary nutrition. Patients with jejunocolic anastomoses may not require supplementary fluids and may only need supplementary nutrition if they have <50 cm residual bowel. Suitable preparations need to be made to ensure adequate facilities for the administration of parenteral nutrition at home; this is formulated and administered according to standard regimens. Particular attention needs to be paid to the vitamin and trace element status of these patients. For example, those who have lost more than 60 cm of ileum require vitamin B_{12} replacement, and selenium deficiency is a particular risk in patients with a jejunostomy.

It is important that the content of the diet is chosen to maximise absorption. The choice should be made according to the nature of the remaining bowel. In patients with an intact colon, a high carbohydrate, low fat diet tends to be beneficial, as complex carbohydrate-containing fibre can be fermented to short chain fatty acids by colonic bacteria and absorbed. However, such a diet involves eating a large volume of food and it may predispose to essential fatty acid deficiency, although sunflower oil can be applied to the skin to prevent this.

FLUID AND ELECTROLYTES

For patients who are net secretors, management includes providing adequate fluid intake and treatment to prevent loss via the jejunostomy. Jejunal loss via a stoma may be up to 4 L/24 h (containing 100 mmol/L of sodium). This degree of fluid and sodium loss stimulates thirst but, because of the nature of the jejunal mucosa, if a solution with a sodium content of less than 90 mmol/L is consumed, there is net movement of sodium from the plasma to the bowel lumen, leading to further intestinal losses. Discouraging intake of hypotonic oral fluids and encouraging intake of an electrolyte mixture is advantageous; a suitable fluid is St Mark's solution, which has a sodium concentration of 90 mmol/L, 60 mmol as sodium chloride and 30 mmol as sodium bicarbonate. This solution also contains 110 mmol/L glucose, as glucose and sodium absorption in the jejunum are coupled. For patients with residual ileum, there is no need for glucose in oral rehydration solution, as ileal water absorption is not affected by the presence of glucose.

Magnesium deficiency can be marked, particularly in patients with an end jejunostomy. Dehydration and sodium depletion lead to secondary hyper-aldosteronism, resulting in renal magnesium loss, exacerbating the effects of gastrointestinal magnesium loss. Oral magnesium replacement tends to exacerbate diarrhoea, and intravenous or subcutaneous replacement may be required. Acidosis can occur secondarily to loss of bicarbonate in gastrointestinal secretions. This should be corrected by adding bicarbonate to parenteral nutrition fluids in the form of acetate, or by giving bicarbonate orally.

DRUG THERAPY

Drugs can be used as a further way to decrease jejunostomy output. Gastric secretions, for example, can be reduced by H_2-receptor antagonists and proton pump inhibitors. As secretions are increased after eating, anti-secretory drugs should be administered before meals. Anti-motility agents such as loperamide and codeine can also be effective.

The remaining bowel can increase its absorptive capacity (adaptation) by various mechanisms, including alterations in hormone secretion and intestinal dimensions and villous hypertrophy. Octreotide, while useful as a somatostatin analogue to decrease gastrointestinal secretions, may affect the production of other gastrointestinal hormones, thereby lessening the potential for adaptation. Growth hormone promotes adaptation and has a role in therapy, particularly in patients being weaned from parenteral nutrition.

Cholestyramine therapy may be useful to bind bile salts if the presence of un-absorbed bile salts in the colon is thought to be contributing to diarrhoea. Pancreatic enzyme supplements may be helpful in selected patients in whom the effects of surgery have compromised the delivery of pancreatic secretions.

Complications

DRUG ABSORPTION

The absorption of many drugs is impaired in SBS, such that either increased oral doses or alternative routes of administration (e.g. intravenous or sublingual administration) are required. Intraindividual variation can make the choice of an accurate dose difficult.

RENAL STONES

Patients with SBS with an intact colon have a 25% risk of developing calcium oxalate renal stones. In health, calcium binds to oxalate in the gut, forming non-absorbable calcium oxalate. In SBS, however, malabsorption of free fatty acids leads to an increase in their binding to calcium, resulting in increased free oxalate, which is absorbed in the colon and subsequently excreted by the kidneys. Stone formation may be exacerbated by dehydration, secondary to high stomal losses, and by hypocitraturia, because of systemic acidosis and hypomagnesaemia (citrate prevents stone nucleation). The management of renal stones includes limiting dietary oxalate, which for those on an oral diet includes reducing intake of rhubarb, nuts, chocolate, tea and strawberries, and increasing calcium intake.

GALLSTONES

Gallstones are common in patients with SBS, occurring in about 45% of both types, and in men more commonly than women. Their composition is usually calcium bilirubinate and they are formed secondarily to gall bladder stasis. Exacerbating factors include rapid weight loss, octreotide therapy and changes in the gut microflora. Prophylactic measures include provision of small amounts of enteral feed to provoke the secretion of cholecystokinin and stimulate gall bladder contraction, or its therapeutic administration. Non-steroidal anti-inflammatory drugs may be effective by altering the glycoproteins required for nucleation.

D-LACTIC ACIDOSIS

D-Lactic acidosis is a rare complication in patients with short bowel syndrome and an intact colon, occurring particularly in those without an ileocaecal valve. It occurs as a result of the absorption of D-lactate produced in the colon by bacterial fermentation of carbohydrate. Initial symptoms include ataxia, blurred vision and nystagmus; confusion can occur and may progress to unconsciousness. The condition is characterised biochemically by a high anion gap metabolic acidosis. Because it is usually the L(+) lactate isomer that is measured in the laboratory (using L(+) lactate dehydrogenase), the condition may remain undetected unless the D(-) lactate isomer is specifically tested for by substituting D(-) standard and D(-) lactate dehydrogenase. The D(-) lactate isomer is normally only present at very low concentrations in plasma.

Intestinal transplantation

The majority of patients with SBS have a normal BMI and undertake normal daily activities. However, their quality of life is often poor owing to problems related to malodorous diarrhoea, the need for frequent emptying of jejunostomy bags and the constraints of administering TPN at home.

Small bowel transplantation is a treatment option in a selected group of patients with irreversible intestinal failure. However, owing to the high risk of associated morbidity and mortality, it is currently restricted to patients with irreversible SBS who have developed life-threatening complications (Figure 7.2).

Indications for intestinal transplantation
Overt or impending liver failure
Limited central venous access
Multiple line infections
Frequent episodes of severe dehydration

Figure 7.2 Indications for intestinal transplantation

Transplantation may be of the intestine alone, of the intestine and liver or of multiple viscera. Transplantation of isolated intestine is performed in patients in whom pathology is limited to the small intestine. Hepato-intestinal transplantation is indicated in patients with failure of both organs, often as a result of TPN-induced liver damage. Multiple visceral transplantation, for example involving stomach, duodenum, pancreas and small intestine, is possible in patients with pathology involving multiple organs, such as extensive vascular thrombosis, although the underlying process should be investigated and treated prior to operation.

Donors should be matched for ABO-compatibility; a small size graft is preferable as the abdominal cavity of recipients is often contracted. Surgery is technically demanding, particularly in patients who have had previous extensive surgery for their underlying condition. Lifelong immunosuppression is required postoperatively. At least 50% survival at five years has been reported after intestinal transplantation.

Functional foods and nutraceuticals

Some foods confer specific health benefits in addition to providing nutrition; these are termed functional foods. Nutraceuticals also have health-promoting effects; they are dietary supplements containing a concentrated form of a bioactive substance that is normally present in food but in a non-food matrix. In some countries, the term 'dietary supplement' is used in preference to nutraceutical. Some countries further classify a nutraceutical as containing many bioactive substances and a nutriceutical as containing a nutrient with a single beneficial effect.

It is difficult to produce a universal definition of functional foods, nutraceuticals and dietary supplements, in part because of the variations in terminology resulting from differences in food and drug regulations between countries. The marketing concept of a functional food is one that states a health claim on the packaging. However, it may be advantageous to market a substance as a food supplement without health claims, in order to avoid the need for it to be licensed as a medicine. Increased regulation is proposed in these areas.

Functional foods

Various functional foods exist and they can be classified according to their content. Figure 7.3 shows some examples of the different types of functional foods available. These are discussed briefly below: the interested reader should consult the references in the Further Reading section for more information.

OAT BRAN FIBRE

Fibre is the component of the diet that is resistant to digestion. Oat bran fibre has been shown to be useful in the management of cardiovascular disease by reducing LDL cholesterol, probably via increasing bile acid secretion and interfering with bile acid reabsorption. Consumption of fibre has been linked to a decreased incidence of colon cancer. Possible mechanisms include increased resistance of intestinal epithelium to the effects of carcinogens secondary to its obtaining nutrition from short chain fatty acids produced by fermentation of fibre in the colon, and decreased intestinal transit time, which reduces opportunities for potential carcinogens to make contact with the gut wall.

OMEGA-3 FATTY ACIDS

Omega-3 fatty acids are found mainly in fish oils and there is evidence that suggests that they may reduce the risk of coronary heart disease. Any effect is likely to be multifactorial, and the mechanisms proposed include alterations in lipid metabolism and cytokine and prostaglandin synthesis.

PLANT STANOLS AND STEROLS

Plant stanols and sterols are marketed principally as constituents of spreading fats and yoghurts. They are similar in structure to cholesterol and act as competitive inhibitors of cholesterol absorption in the small intestine, thereby reducing plasma LDL cholesterol. Plant sterols may also have a protective effect with regard to cancer risk, particularly for prostate and colon cancers.

SOY PROTEIN

Soy protein can bring about a decrease in LDL cholesterol and hence reduce cardiovascular risk. Hypotheses for the cause of this effect propose that its amino acid composition, which has a low ratio of lysine to arginine, may be responsible for increased insulin release, which then affects cholesterol synthesis, lipoprotein

---

Functional foods classified by content

Basic foods
 Bran cereal

Processed food
 Calcium-enriched fruit juices

Food enriched by traditional methods/genetic engineering to increase a specific functional component
 Oat bran with increased β-glucan
 Tomatoes with increased lycopene

Isolated purified preparations of active ingredients in food form
 Omega-3 fatty acids from fish oil
 Soy protein
 Stanols
 Pre- pro- and synbiotics

Figure 7.3 Functional foods classified by content

clearance and biliary cholesterol excretion. Soy protein also contains oestrogen-like isoflavonoids, which have multiple effects, including acting as antioxidants and influencing thrombus formation and vascular reactivity.

PROBIOTICS

Probiotics are live microbial food supplements: the most commonly available preparations contain *Lactobacilli, Streptococci* and *Bifidobacteria*, which are major components of the normal gut environment. In order to be an effective probiotic, the bacteria contained in the food need to be resistant to the effects of gastric acid, digestion by pancreatic enzymes and to the detergent properties of bile. Most companies that market probiotics and groups undertaking research into these foods have tended to favour yoghurt and fermented milk drinks as probiotic sources. Other sources do exist, for example, hard cheese, soy sauce and gherkins, but their potential is largely uninvestigated.

Multiple actions have been proposed to account for the health benefits of probiotics. These include competitive inhibition preventing the attachment of gut pathogens to the gastrointestinal epithelium, the secretion by probiotics of metabolites such as certain amino acids that have inhibitory actions and lead to increased mucus secretion, and the effects of probiotics on the immune response.

Little is known about the optimum dosage required. If competitive inhibition at bacterial adhesion sites is essential to the mode of action, then the dose will be dependent on relative affinity; other factors could include source, co-administration with food, gastric pH and gut motility.

PREBIOTICS

Prebiotics are nondigestible food ingredients that beneficially affect the host by selectively stimulating the growth or activity of one or a limited number of bacterial species in the colon, usually (but not exclusively) *Lactobacilli* and *Bifidobacteria*. Currently available prebiotics are carbohydrates, for example inulin and synthetic fructo-oligosaccharides. They are not significantly absorbed in the small intestine but undergo fermentation in the colon; it is the resulting short chain fatty acids that bring about their positive effect. Beneficial effects attributed to prebiotics include alteration of lipid metabolism, manifest as a reduction in fasting triglyceride concentration, and a decreased fasting insulin concentration. Other suggested effects are increased absorption of calcium and an inhibitory effect on carcinogenesis.

Probiotics have a transient function and regular daily consumption is needed to sustain their effect. Prebiotics encourage growth of natural bowel flora and may, therefore, have a more long-lasting effect.

SYNBIOTICS

Synbiotics contain probiotics and prebiotics, the prebiotic selectively favouring the conditions that are optimal for the action of the probiotic. While benefits have been documented, there are theoretical risks associated with probiotic use, in particular microbial resistance and detrimental immune modulation. Probiotic use has been reported to be associated with sepsis, especially in high risk groups such as neonates and the immune compromised.

Nutraceuticals

A large number of nutraceuticals and dietary supplements are available commercially although evidence for efficacy is not available for many (Figure 7.4). Individual vitamins and trace elements have been discussed in Chapter 2.

Nutraceuticals are taken for pharmaceutical benefit or to correct deficiency. As marketing is targeted at the general public, the focus tends to be on diseases of high prevalence. A large number are available via shops and the internet, but only the most common, which have been evaluated in clinical trials, are discussed here.

Nutraceuticals and dietary supplements

Vitamins

Trace elements

Herbs/botanicals

Amino acids

Metabolites

Tissue extracts

Figure 7.4 Nutraceuticals and dietary supplements

CARDIOVASCULAR DISEASE

Consumption of garlic has been shown to be associated with a reduction in total and LDL cholesterol and triglyceride concentrations. One proposed mechanism is inhibition of the enzyme HMGCoA reductase. Its active agent is thought to be allicin, which is released on crushing and is destroyed by cooking; a large variation in effect has been shown between different commercial extracts. Ginger, capsaicin and curcumin have also been shown to favourably influence lipid profiles in rat models.

MUSCULOSKELETAL DISEASE

A number of nutraceuticals are promoted for use in arthritis, and of these there is evidence available supporting the use of glucosamine and chondroitin sulphate. Glucosamine is a precursor of glucosaminoglycan and has a beneficial effect on the production of articular cartilage and the nature of synovial fluid. Chondroitin sulphate is a component of cartilage that, when taken orally, has been shown to improve symptoms and may have a structural effect. When administered together, the effects of glucosamine and chondroitin sulphate are synergistic.

Ginger has anti-inflammatory properties through its inhibition of arachidonic acid metabolism, but it has been shown to have only a minor effect as an analgesic in arthritis.

Creatine supplementation has been demonstrated to improve muscle performance in athletes, although not all show a response, and this may be because not all are deficient. Creatine is present in the diet, particularly in meat and fish, and can be synthesised in muscle, kidney and pancreas. It is stored predominantly in muscle, where its interconversion to phosphocreatine by creatine kinase is linked to the production of ATP, particularly for short, high energy activity. It is of particular importance to clinical biochemists as its presence in excess in plasma may cause positive interference in enzymatic creatinine assays that detect creatine hydrolysed from creatinine by creatininase.

PSYCHOLOGICAL DISORDERS

Several nutraceuticals have been shown to be of use in treating psychological disorders, including passionflower, which has been shown to be an effective sedative, and valerian, which is widely used to treat anxiety. St John's Wort (*Hypericum perforatum*) in particular has received much attention, especially as a treatment for depression; it is of proven value in mild to moderate depression but there is insufficient evidence to assess its effect in severe depression. Its active components, hypericin and hyperforin, act to inhibit the reuptake of serotonin, dopamine and noradrenaline and to activate γ-aminobenzoic acid and glutamate receptors. As it induces cytochrome P450, it can interfere with the metabolism of prescribed and over-the-counter drugs, for example decreasing the effects of warfarin and oral contraceptives. Therefore, enquiry about the use of functional foods and nutraceuticals should be a routine part of clinical history taking.

It may be that nutraceuticals act to correct deficiencies in some patients who benefit from taking them. Recommended daily allowances (RDA) for vitamins and trace elements are derived from population data but these may underestimate the requirements of some individuals. In addition, these requirements may change without any corresponding changes in dietary intake, for example, as a result of intensive physical exercise and in individuals taking medication.

Excessive quantities of dietary supplements can be toxic and certain populations can be particularly susceptible, e.g. large doses of vitamin E and carotenoids may be associated with an increased risk of lung cancer in smokers. Nutriomic research may lead to the identification of measurable indicators that can be easily applied to the population to enable the appropriate use of these and other dietary components.

Nutriomics and nutrigenetics

Nutriomics and nutrigenetics are concerned with examining the interface between nutrition and cellular and genetic processes. Nutrigenetics identifies and characterises gene variants associated with differing responses to nutrients. Nutriomics makes use of genetic tools to investigate a biological system following a nutritional stimulus and seeks to explain how nutrients are able to regulate gene expression.

Various '-omic' terms are used to describe the techniques involved. Transcriptomics uses microarrays to analyse gene expression by studying mRNA. Proteomics investigates protein expression, often by using separation on two-dimensional gels, followed by mass spectrometric techniques for identification. Metabolomics examines the response of metabolites in cells or body fluids to particular nutrients, using methodologies such as chromatography or liquid chromatography in combination with mass spectrometry and nuclear magnetic resonance.

It has been clear for some time that dietary modification can alter the course of some monogenic diseases, for example phenylketonuria and galactosaemia. Nutrigenetics is now demonstrating how it may be possible to provide more specific nutritional advice for patients with polygenic disorders. For example, with respect to cardiovascular disorders, individuals with a polymorphism in the *APO1* gene promoter region show a particularly favourable response in plasma HDL concentration to dietary polyunsaturated fatty acids, whereas obese individuals with a specific polymorphism in lipoprotein lipase show marked improvements in their lipid profiles with just a low calorie diet.

Nutriomics and nutrigenetics are revealing the complexity of the relationship between nutrition and the genome but are also providing potential opportunities to optimise the way in which nutritional interventions are used. In the future, it may be possible to refine recommendations on nutritional requirements taking into account both genetic background and individual physiology, and to devise personalised dietary regimens to minimise and manage disease.

Further reading

Avenell A. Glutamine in critical care: current evidence from systematic reviews. Proc Nutr Soc 2006; **65:** 236-241.

Dellinger RP, Carlet JM, Masur H, Gulak H, Calandra T *et al.* for the Surviving Sepsis Campaign Management Guidelines Committee. Surviving sepsis campaign guidelines for the management of severe sepsis and septic shock. Crit Care Med 2004; **32:** 858-873.

Hadley JS, Hinds CJ. Anabolic strategies in critical illness. Curr Opin Pharmacol 2003; **2:** 700-707.

Three reviews discussing potentially beneficial interventions in critical care patients.

Mann J. Cardiovascular disease. In: Geissler C, Powers H. Human Nutrition. Edinburgh: Churchill Livingstone, 2005, pp 363-378.

Mitch WE, Walser M. Nutritional therapy in renal disease. In: Brenner BM (ed). Brenner and Rector's The Kidney (7th edition). Philadelphia, USA: Saunders, 2004, pp2491-2538.

Morgan MY. Nutritional aspects of liver and biliary disease. In: Bircher J, Benhamun J-P, McIntyre N, Rizzetto M, Rodés J (eds). Oxford Textbook of Clinical Hepatology (2nd edition). Oxford: Oxford University Press; 1999, pp 1923-1981.

Detailed accounts of nutritional interventions in cardiovascular, renal and hepatic disease, respectively.

Buckman AL. Etiology and initial management of short bowel syndrome. Gastroenterol 2006; **130 (Suppl 1):** S5-S15.
This supplement contains several other useful reviews of nutrition-related topics.

Elliott R, Ong TJ. Nutritional genomics. Brit Med J 2002; **324:** 1438-1442.
This short review considers the scope and implications of other nutritionally related '-omics' in addition to genomics.

Halstead CH. Dietary supplements and functional foods: 2 sides of a coin. Am J Clin Nutr 2003; **77 (Suppl 4):** 1001S-1007S.
A review of the topic that considers the patient's persepectives as well as the health professional's.

Gibney MJ, Walsh M, Brennan L, Roche HM, German B, van Ommen B. Metabolomics in human nutrition: opportunities and challenges. Am J Clin Nutr 2005; **82:** 497-503.

Nightingale JM. Management of patients with a short bowel. World J Gastroenterol 2001; **7:** 741-751.